THE ANTI-INFLAMMATORY DIET COOKBOOK

Meal Prep Made Simple For Beginners

S.L. Mills

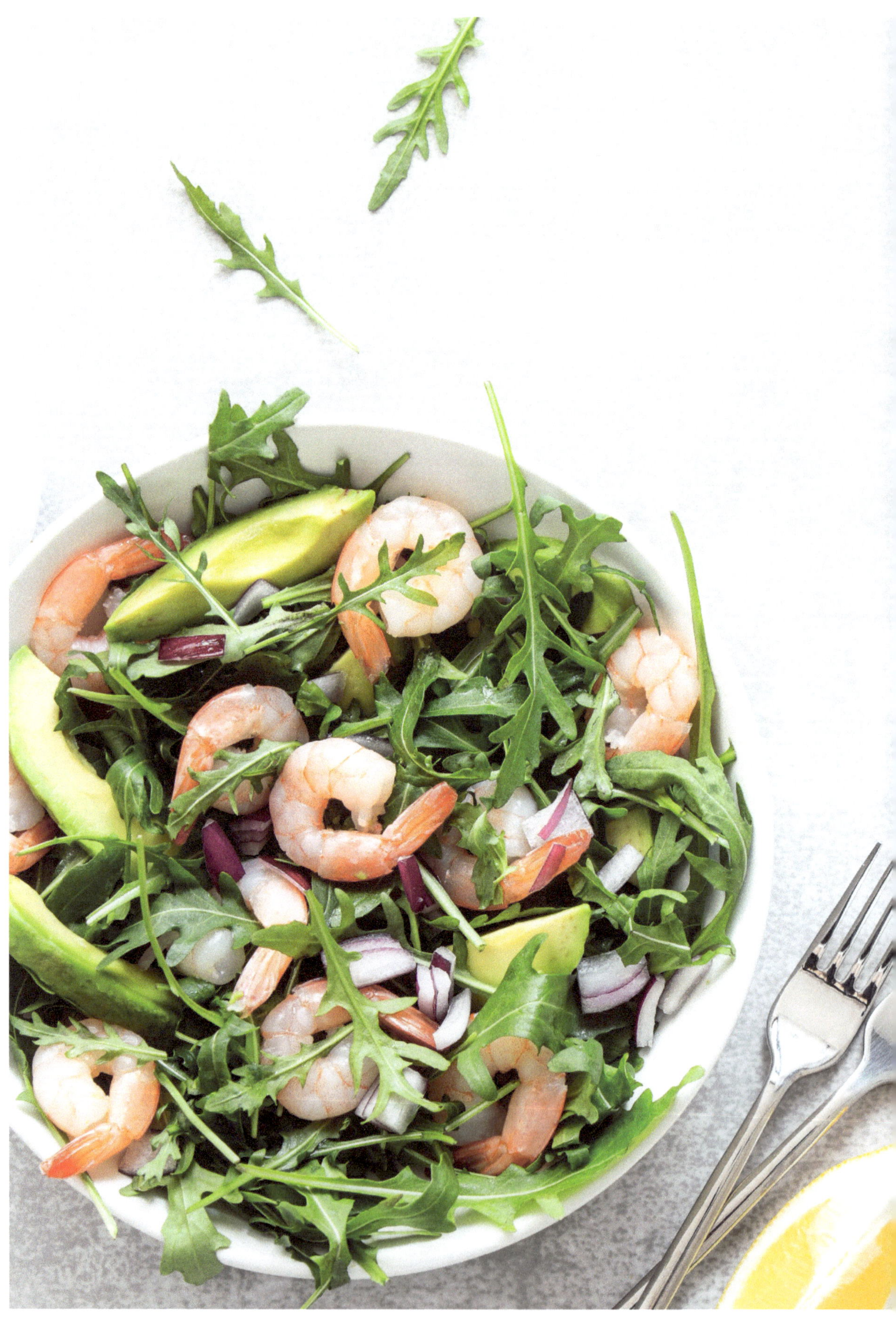

About Me

I work in the healthcare field as an educator. I love great food and I found that the right foods can help bring a balance to our physical, mental and emotional well being. Inflammation and the foods we choose impacts in ways that can not be underestimated. This book is a labor of love for me. Polycystic ovarian syndrome, heart and kidney disease have touched people I hold very precious in my life. These conditions inspired me to provide good, comforting meals that could help with managing good anti- inflammatory diet. I wanted to create recipes that not only would be flavorful but healthy as well.

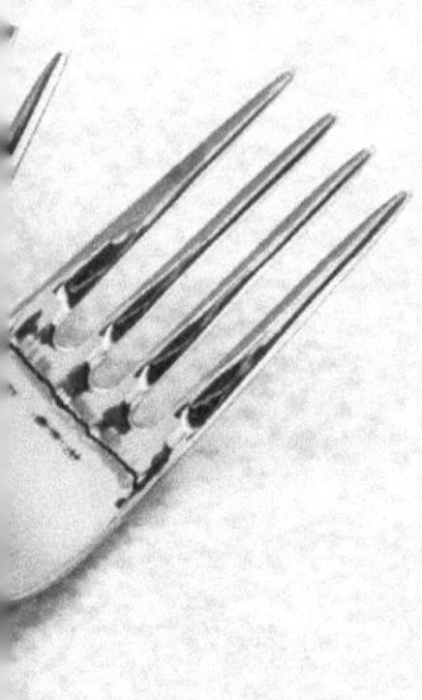

Disclaimer: General Food Safety Disclaimer The reader assumes full responsibility for using their best judgment when cooking with raw ingredients such as beef, poultry, or eggs, and seeking information from an official food safety authority if they are unsure. The reader must also take care to not physically injure themselves by coming into contact with hot surfaces, sharp blades, and other kitchen hazards. It is the responsibility of the reader to review all listed ingredients in a recipe before cooking to ensure that none of the ingredients may cause a potential adverse reactions.

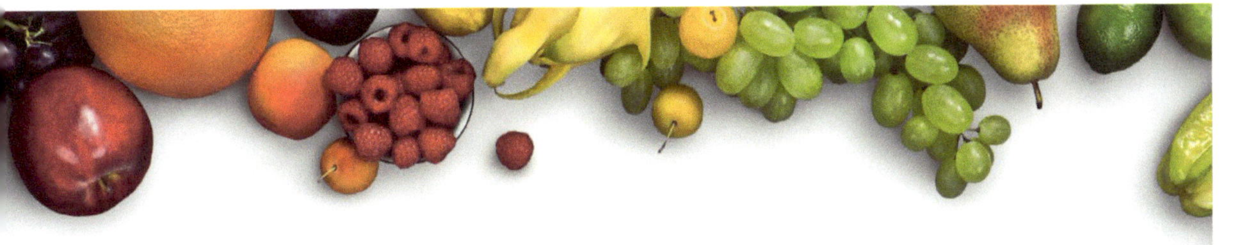

Contents

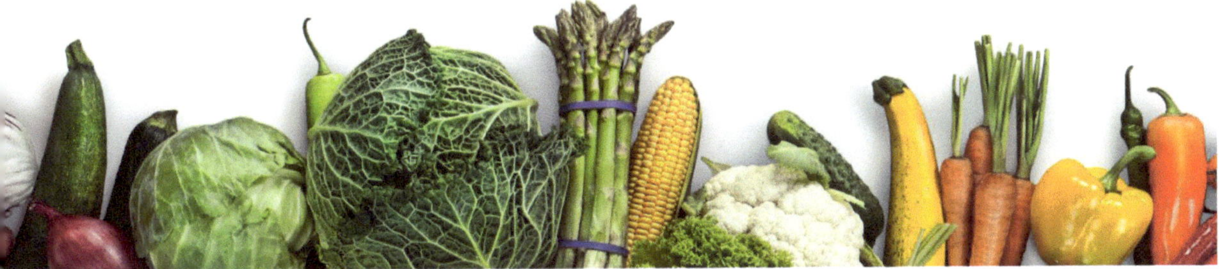

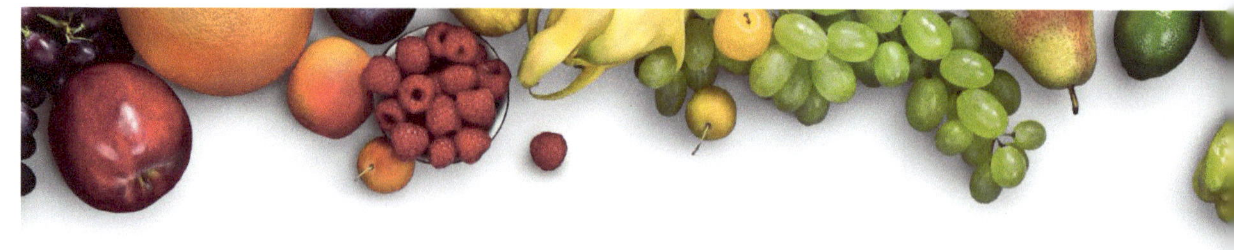

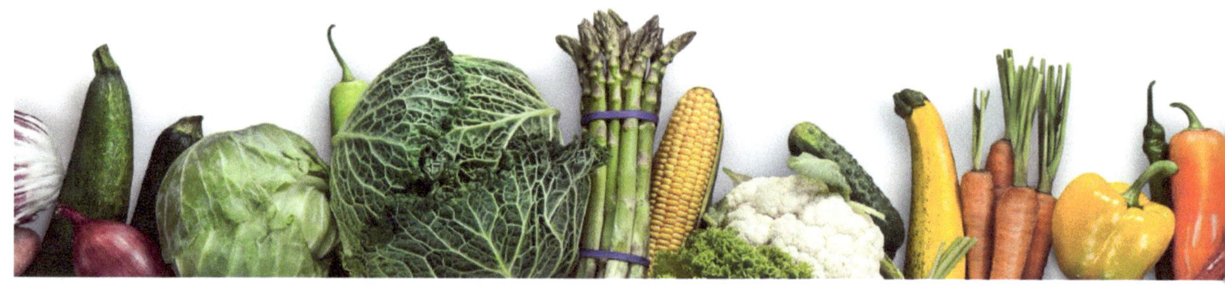

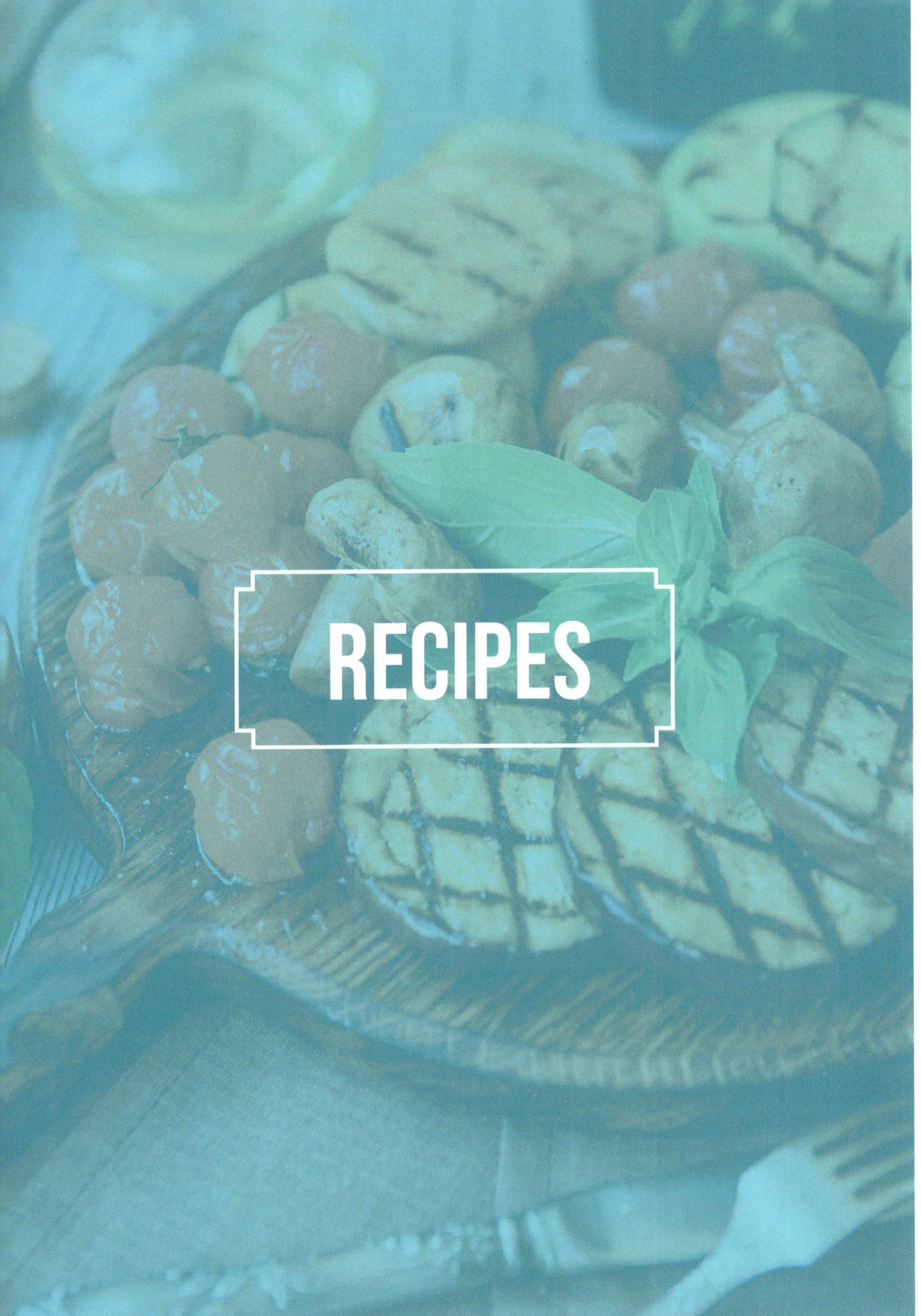
RECIPES

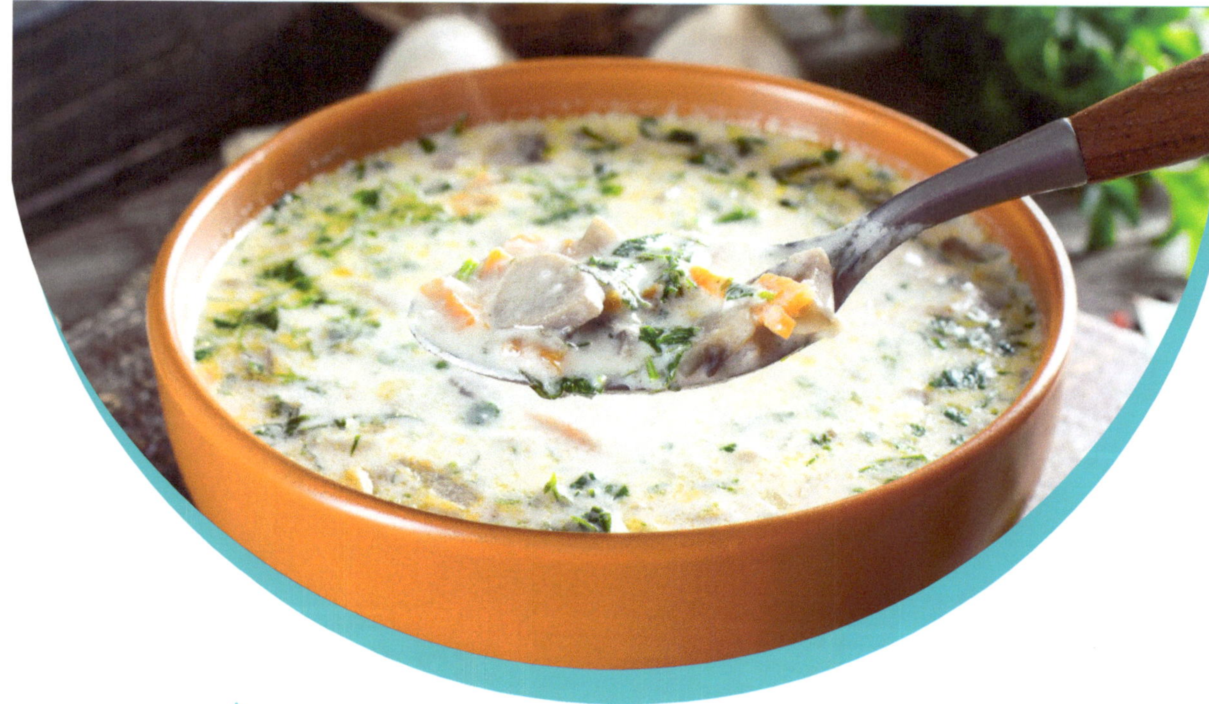

SPINCREAMY CHICKEN AND MUSHROOM SOUP

**Total Time:
20 Mins**

**Serving:
2**

Ingredients

2 tablespoons unsalted butter
1 onion, chopped
2 cloves garlic, minced
8 oz mushrooms, sliced
1 teaspoon dried thyme
4 cups low-sodium chicken broth
2 cups of low-fat milk
1 lb cooked chicken breast, shredded
Salt and pepper to taste

Directions

1. In a large pot, melt butter over medium heat.
2. Add onion and garlic, and cook until onion is translucent about 5 minutes.
3. Add mushrooms and thyme, and cook for another 5 minutes.
4. Add chicken broth and milk, and bring to a simmer.
5. Add chicken breast and cook until heated through about 5 minutes.
6. Season with salt and pepper to taste.

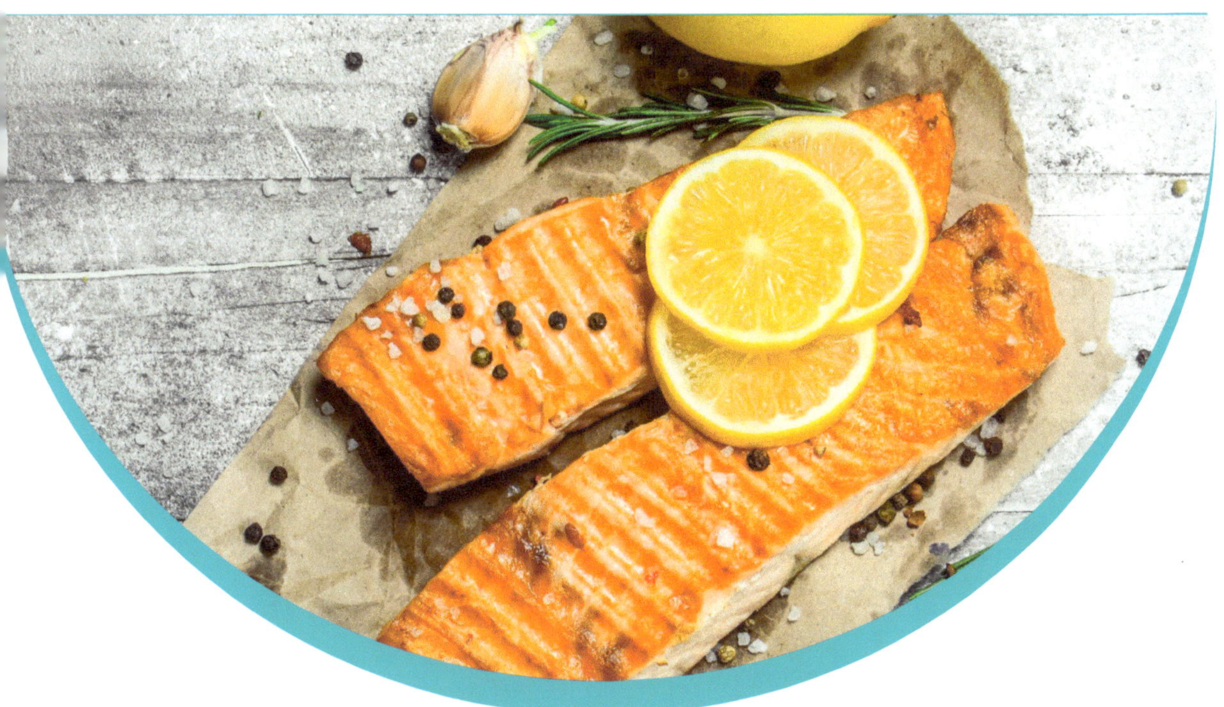

GRILLED LEMON PEPPER SALMON

Total Time:
6 Mins

Serving:
4

Ingredients

4 4-oz salmon fillets
1 tablespoon olive oil
1 lemon, sliced
1 tablespoon black pepper
Salt to taste

Directions

1. Preheat the grill to medium-high heat.
2. Brush salmon fillets with olive oil.
3. Season with black pepper and salt.
4. Place lemon slices on top of salmon fillets.
5. Grill salmon for 4-5 minutes per side or until cooked through.

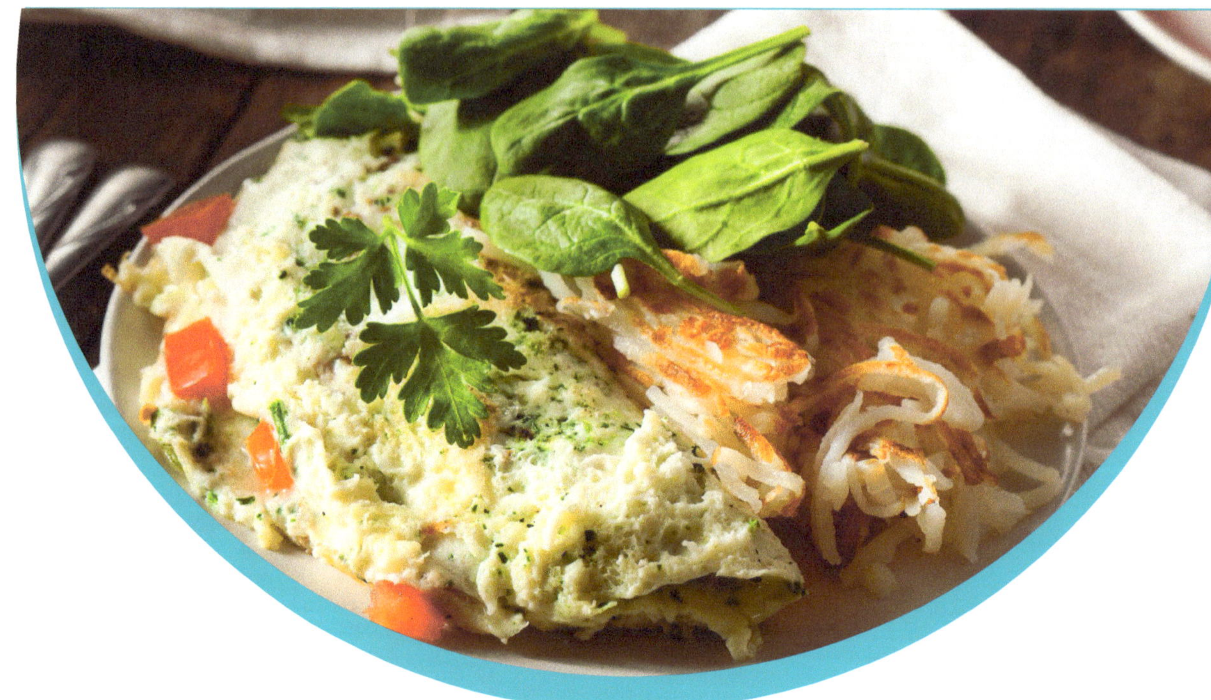

EGG WHITE OMELETE

Total Time:
5 Mins

Serving:
2

Ingredients

4 egg whites
1 teaspoon olive oil
1/4 cup chopped spinach
1/4 cup chopped mushrooms
1/4 cup chopped bell peppers
Salt and pepper to taste

Directions

1. In a small bowl, whisk egg whites with salt and pepper.
2. Heat olive oil in a non-stick pan over medium heat.
3. Add spinach, mushrooms, and bell peppers, and sauté until vegetables are tender.
4. Pour egg whites into the pan and cook for 2-3 minutes, until the bottom is set.
5. Fold the omelet in half and continue cooking for another 1-2 minutes.

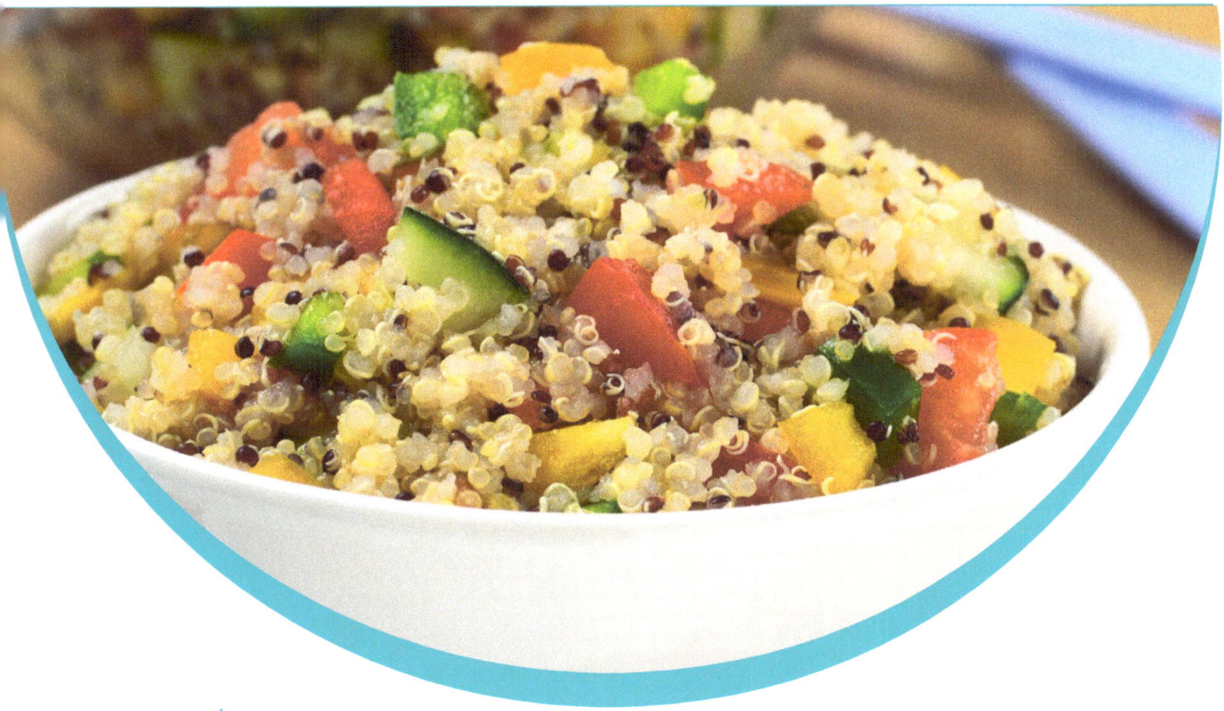

QUINOA SALAD

Ingredients

Total Time:
25 Mins

Serving:
2

1 cup quinoa, rinsed
2 cups water
1/2 cucumber, chopped
1/2 tomato, chopped
1/2 bell pepper, chopped
2 tablespoons chopped parsley
2 tablespoons chopped mint
1/4 cup olive oil

1/4 cup lemon juice
Salt and pepper to taste

Directions

1. In a medium pot, bring quinoa and water to a boil.
2. Reduce heat to low, cover, and simmer for 15-20 minutes, until quinoa is tender and water is absorbed.
3. Mix cooked quinoa, cucumber, tomato, bell pepper, parsley, and mint
4. in a large bowl.
5. Whisk together olive oil, lemon juice, salt, and pepper in a small bowl.
6. Pour dressing over quinoa salad and toss to combine.

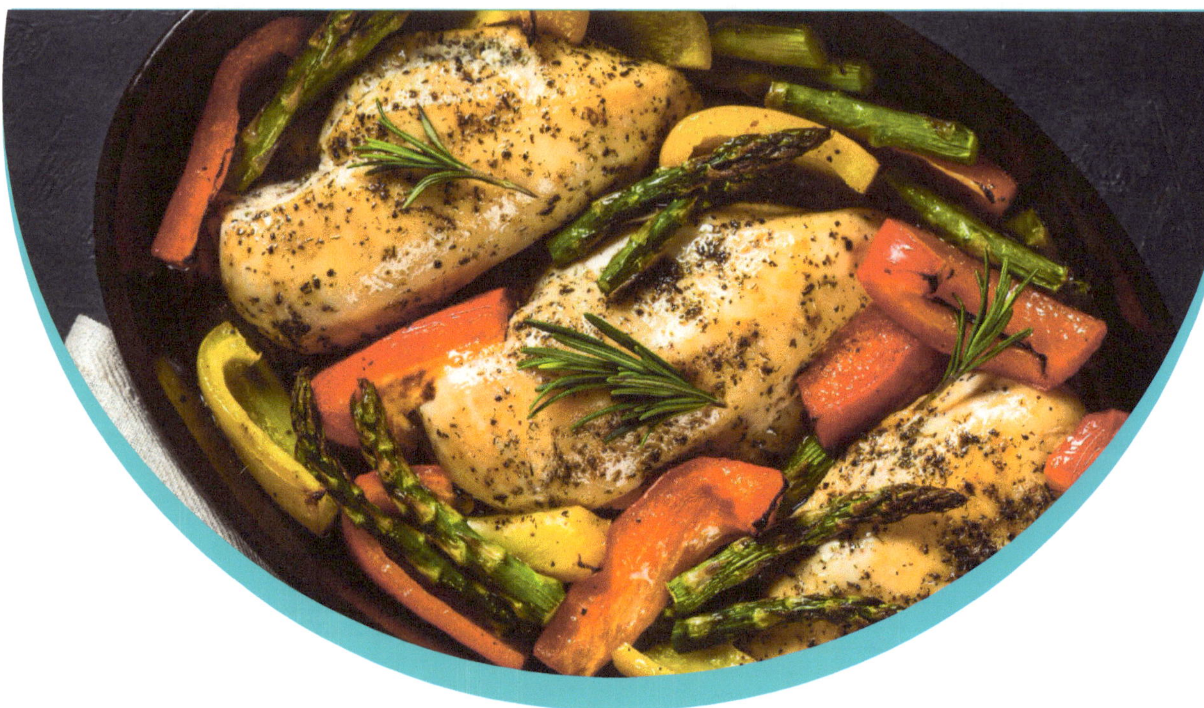

BAKED CHICKEN AND VEGETABLES

Ingredients

Total Time:
30 Mins

Serving:
4

4 boneless, skinless chicken breasts
2 teaspoons low-sodium seasoning
1 teaspoon olive oil
1/2 lb carrots, peeled and chopped
1/2 lb green beans, trimmed
1/2 onion, chopped
Salt and pepper to taste

Directions

1. Preheat oven to 400°F.
2. Season chicken breasts with low-sodium seasoning and salt and pepper to taste.
3. Toss carrots, green beans, and onion with olive oil, salt, and pepper in a large bowl.
4. Arrange chicken breasts in a single layer in a baking dish.
5. Surround the chicken with seasoned vegetables.
6. Bake for 20-25 minutes, until chicken is cooked and vegetables are tender.

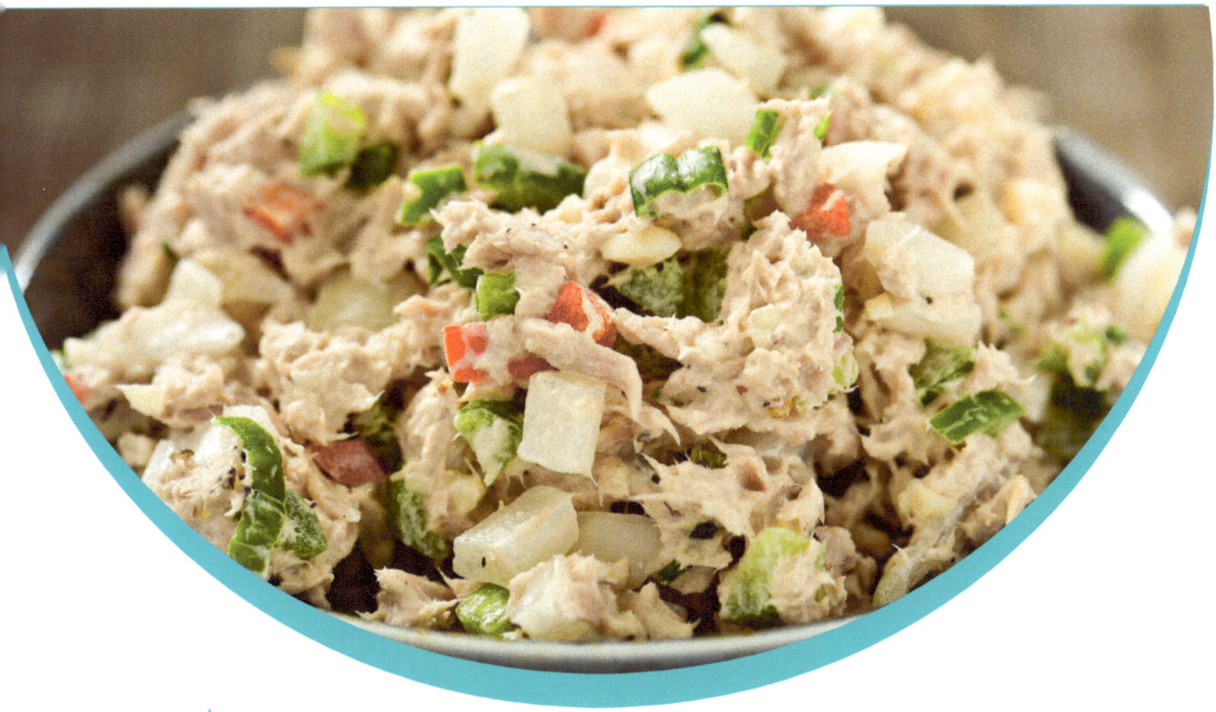

TUNA SALAD WITH GREEK YOGURT

**Total Time:
5 Mins**

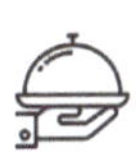

**Serving:
1**

Ingredients

2 cans of tuna, drained
1/2 cup plain Greek yogurt
1/4 cup diced celery
1/4 cup diced red onion
1 tablespoon chopped dill
1 tablespoon lemon juice
Salt and pepper to taste

Directions

1. Mix tuna, Greek yogurt, celery, red onion, dill, lemon juice, salt, and pepper in a medium bowl.
2. Serve over a bed of mixed greens or in a sandwich with whole wheat bread.

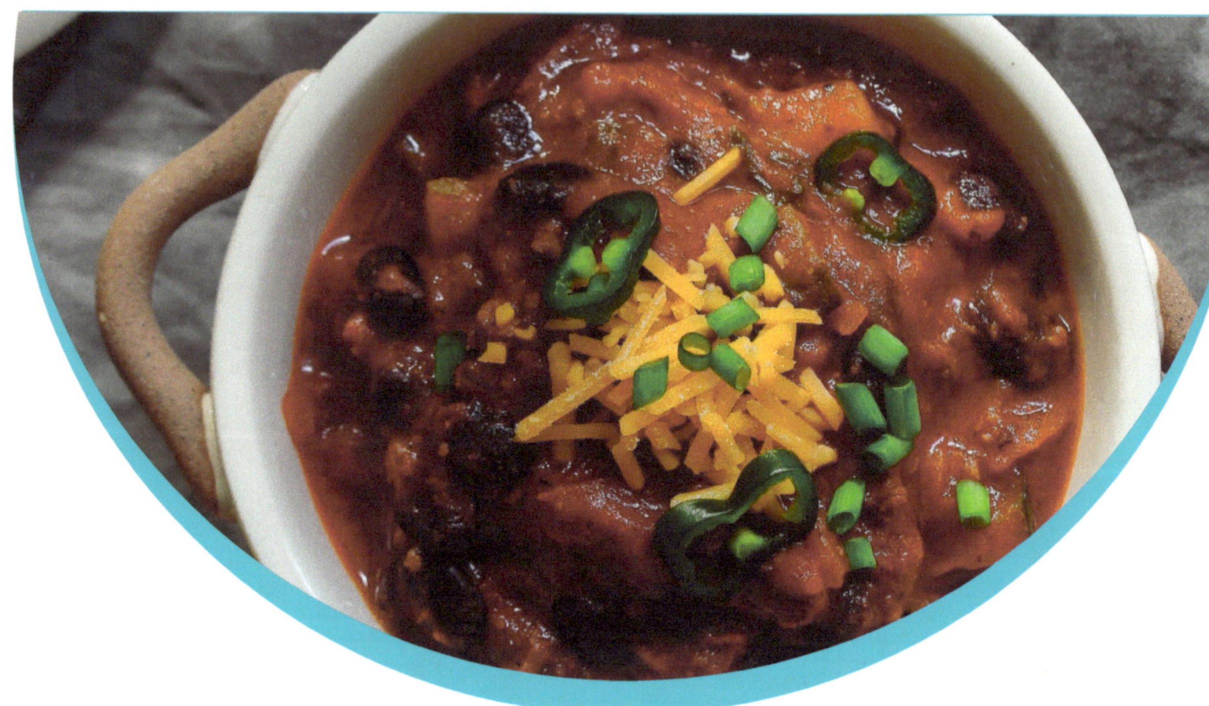

TURKEY CHILI

Total Time:
35 Mins

Serving:
2

Ingredients

1 lb ground turkey
1 onion, chopped
1 red bell pepper, chopped
2 garlic cloves, minced
1 tablespoon chili powder
1 teaspoon ground cumin
1/2 teaspoon smoked paprika
1/4 teaspoon cayenne pepper

2 cups low-sodium chicken broth
1 can kidney beans, drained and rinsed
Salt and pepper to taste

Directions

1. In a large pot, cook ground turkey over medium-high heat until browned.
2. Add onion, bell pepper, and garlic, and cook for 5-7 minutes, until vegetables are tender.
3. Add chili powder, cumin, paprika, and cayenne pepper, and cook for 1-2 minutes, until fragrant.
4. Add chicken broth and kidney beans, and bring to a simmer.
5. Reduce heat to low and let simmer for 15-20 minutes.
6. Season with salt and pepper to taste.

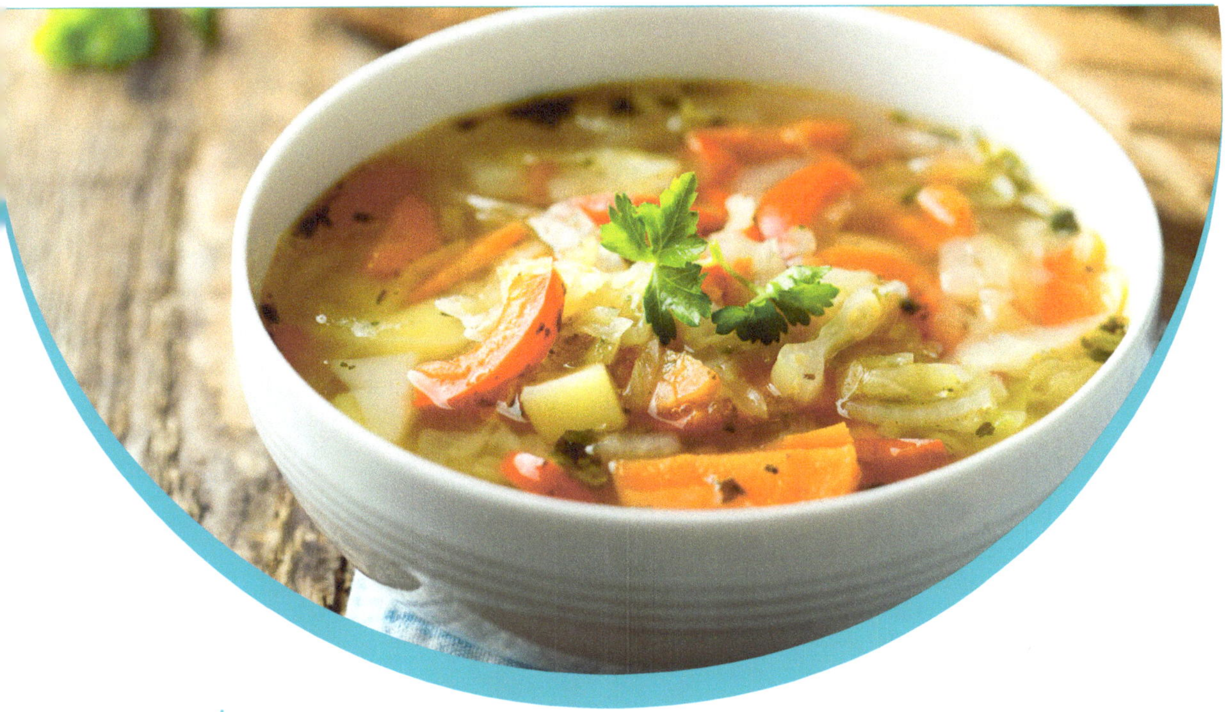

![Low-sodium vegetable soup in a white bowl]

LOW-SODIUM VEGETABLE SOUP

Ingredients

Total Time:
40 Mins

Serving:
2

2 tablespoons olive oil
1 onion, chopped
2 garlic cloves, minced
2 carrots, peeled and chopped
2 celery stalks, chopped
1 zucchini, chopped
1 yellow squash, chopped
4 cups low-sodium vegetable broth

1 can diced tomatoes
1 teaspoon dried thyme
Salt and pepper to taste

Directions

1. In a large pot, heat olive oil over medium heat.
2. Add onion and garlic, and cook until onion is translucent about 5 minutes.
3. Add carrots, celery, zucchini, and yellow squash, and cook for another 5-7 minutes.
4. Add vegetable broth, diced tomatoes, and thyme, and bring to a simmer.
5. Reduce heat to low and let simmer for 15-20 minutes.
6. Season with salt and pepper to taste.

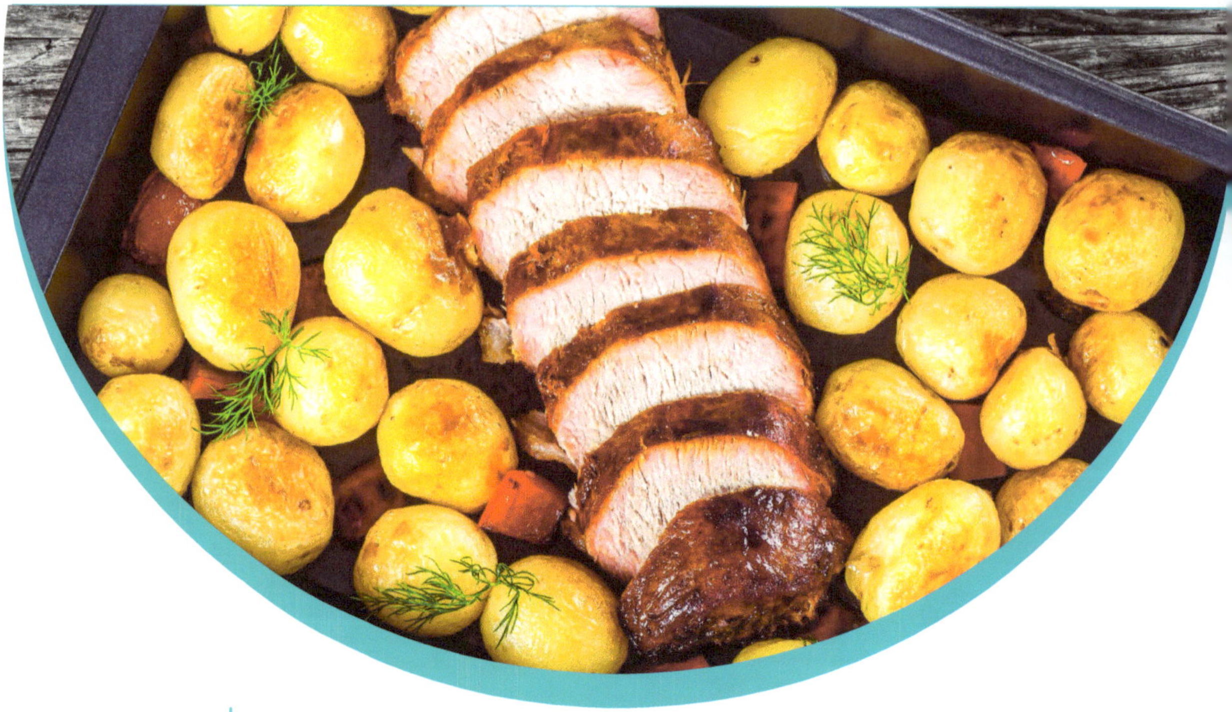

ROASTED PORK TENDERLOIN

Ingredients

**Total Time:
35 Mins**

**Serving:
4**

1 lb pork tenderloin
2 sweet potatoes, peeled and chopped
1 onion, chopped
2 garlic cloves, minced
1 tablespoon olive oil
1 teaspoon dried rosemary
Salt and pepper to taste

Directions

1. Preheat oven to 375°F.
2. Toss sweet potatoes, onion, garlic, olive oil, rosemary, salt, and pepper in a large bowl.
3. Arrange vegetables in a single layer in a baking dish.
4. Season pork tenderloin with salt and pepper and place on top of the vegetables.
5. Roast for 25-30 minutes until pork is cooked and vegetables are tender.

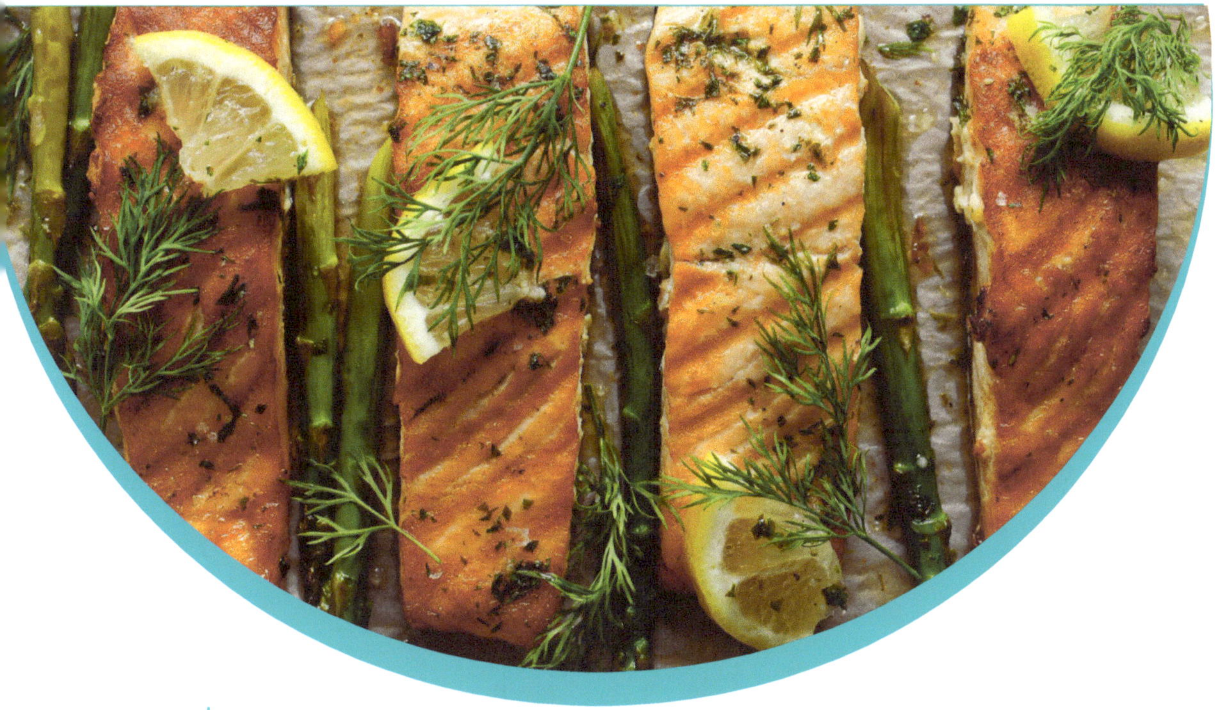

**Total Time:
20 Mins**

**Serving:
4**

BAKED SALMON WITH LEMON AND DILL

Ingredients

4 salmon fillets
2 tablespoons olive oil
2 tablespoons lemon juice
2 tablespoons chopped fresh dill
Salt and pepper to taste

Directions

1. Preheat oven to 375°F.
2. Whisk together olive oil, lemon juice, dill, salt, and pepper in a small bowl.
3. Place salmon fillets on a baking sheet lined with parchment paper.
4. Brush the lemon-dill mixture over the salmon.
5. Bake for 12-15 minutes, until salmon is cooked through.

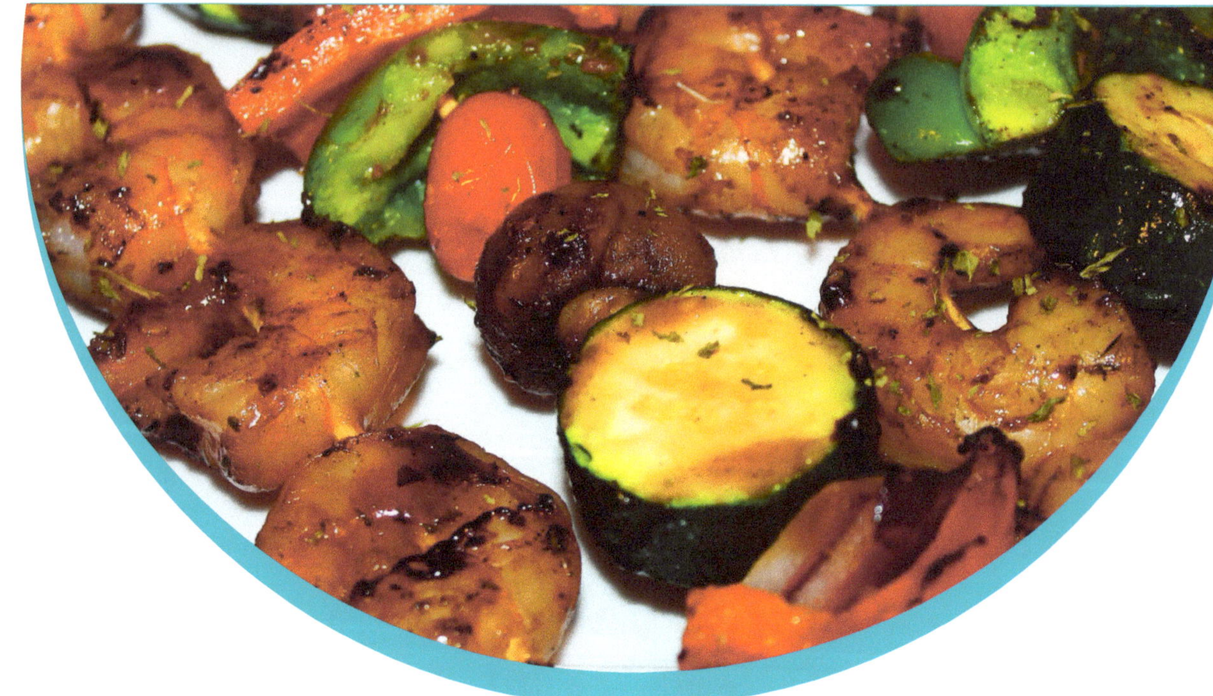

GRILLED SHRIMP SKEWERS WITH VEGETABLES

**Total Time:
10 Mins**

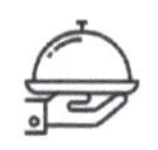

**Serving:
2**

Ingredients

1 lb large shrimp, peeled and deveined
1 red bell pepper, chopped
1 green bell pepper, chopped
1 zucchini, chopped
1 yellow squash, chopped
2 tablespoons olive oil
2 garlic cloves, minced

Salt and pepper to taste

Directions

1. Preheat the grill to medium-high heat.
2. Toss shrimp and vegetables with olive oil, garlic, salt, and pepper in a large bowl.
3. Thread shrimp and vegetables onto skewers.
4. Grill skewers for 2-3 minutes per side until shrimp is pink and cooked through.

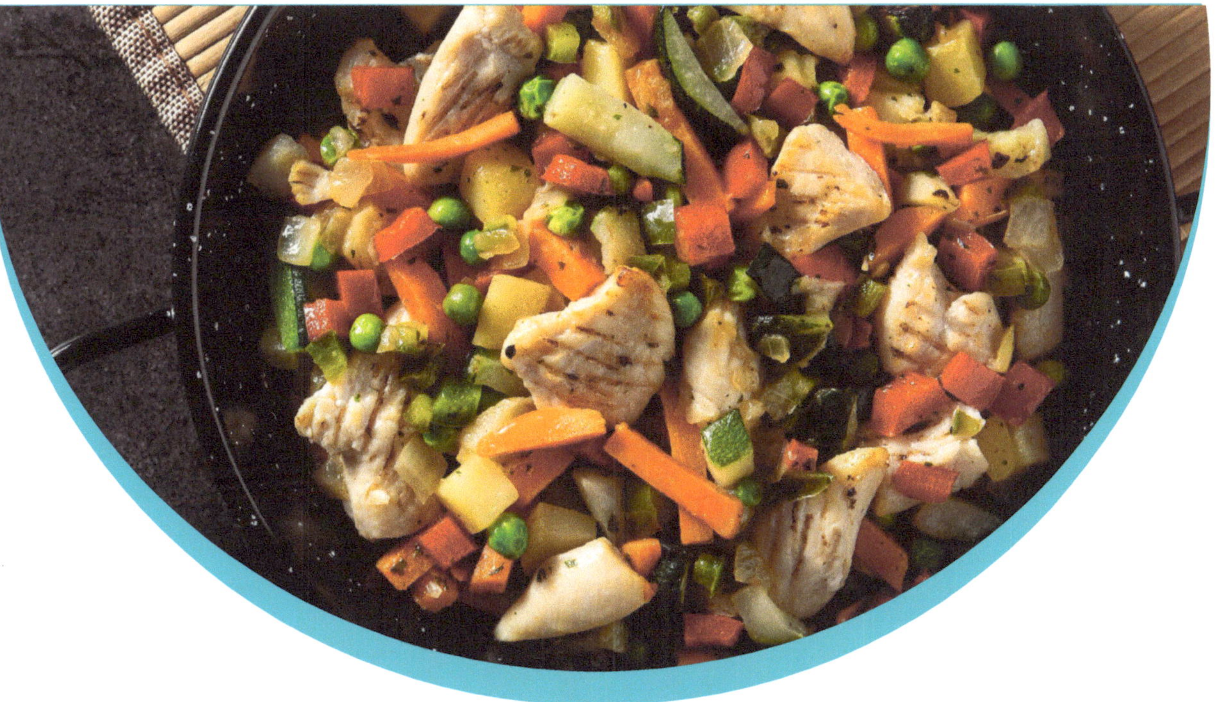

VEGETABLE AND CHICKEN STIR-FRY

Ingredients

**Total Time:
20 Mins**

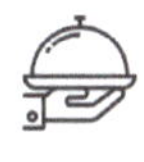

**Serving:
4**

1 lb boneless, skinless chicken breasts, sliced
1 onion, chopped
2 garlic cloves, minced
2 carrots, peeled and chopped
1 red bell pepper, chopped
1 green bell pepper, chopped
1 zucchini, chopped

2 tablespoons olive oil
2 tablespoons low-sodium soy sauce
1 tablespoon cornstarch
Salt and pepper to taste

Directions

1. In a large skillet or wok, heat olive oil over high heat.
2. Add chicken and cook until browned on all sides, about 5 minutes.
3. Add onion, garlic, carrots, and bell peppers, and cook for another 5-7 minutes.
4. Add zucchini and cook for 2-3 minutes, until vegetables are tender.
5. In a small bowl, whisk together soy sauce and cornstarch.
6. Add the soy sauce mixture to the skillet and stir until the sauce thickens.
7. Season with salt and pepper to taste.

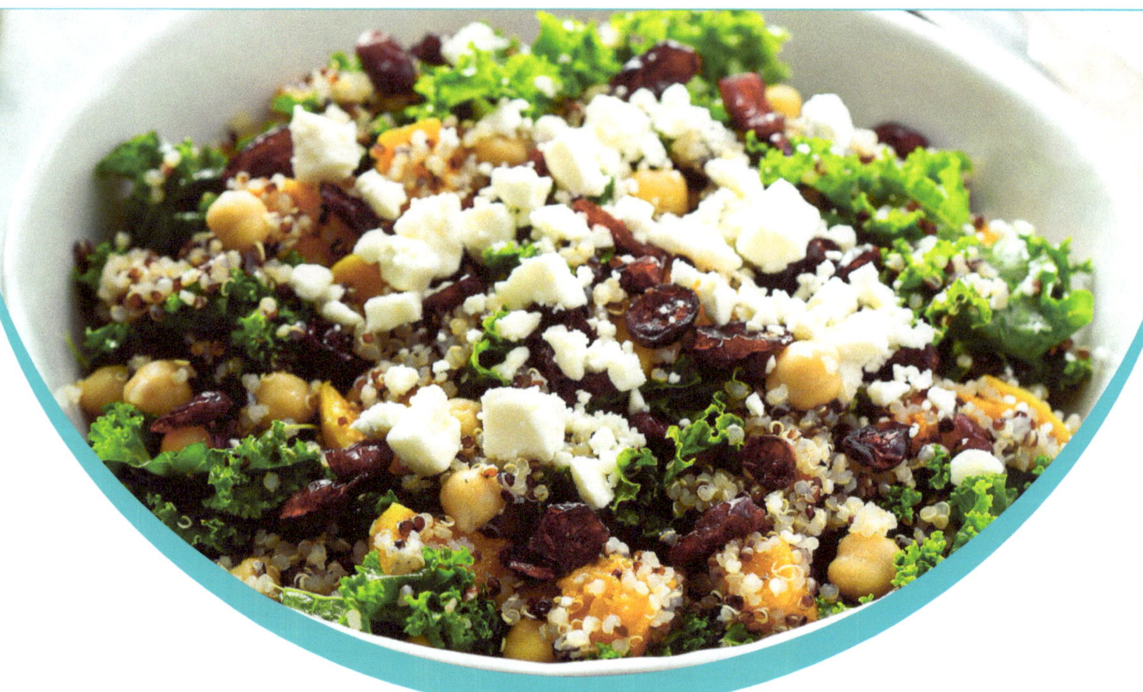

QUINOA SALAD WITH ROASTED VEGETABLES

Ingredients

**Total Time:
55 Mins**

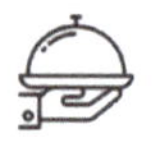

**Serving:
2**

1 cup quinoa
2 cups low-sodium vegetable broth
2 sweet potatoes, peeled and
chopped
1 onion, chopped
1 red bell pepper, chopped
1 tablespoon olive oil
Salt and pepper to taste

Directions

1. Preheat oven to 375°F.
2. In a large bowl, toss sweet potatoes, onion, and red bell pepper with olive oil, salt, and pepper.
3. Arrange vegetables in a single layer on a baking sheet lined with parchment paper.
4. Roast for 25-30 minutes, until vegetables are tender and lightly browned.
5. In a medium pot, bring vegetable broth to a boil.
6. Add quinoa and reduce heat to low.
7. Cover and simmer for 15-20 minutes, until quinoa is cooked and liquid is absorbed.
8. In a large bowl, combine quinoa and roasted vegetables.
9. Season with additional salt and pepper to taste.

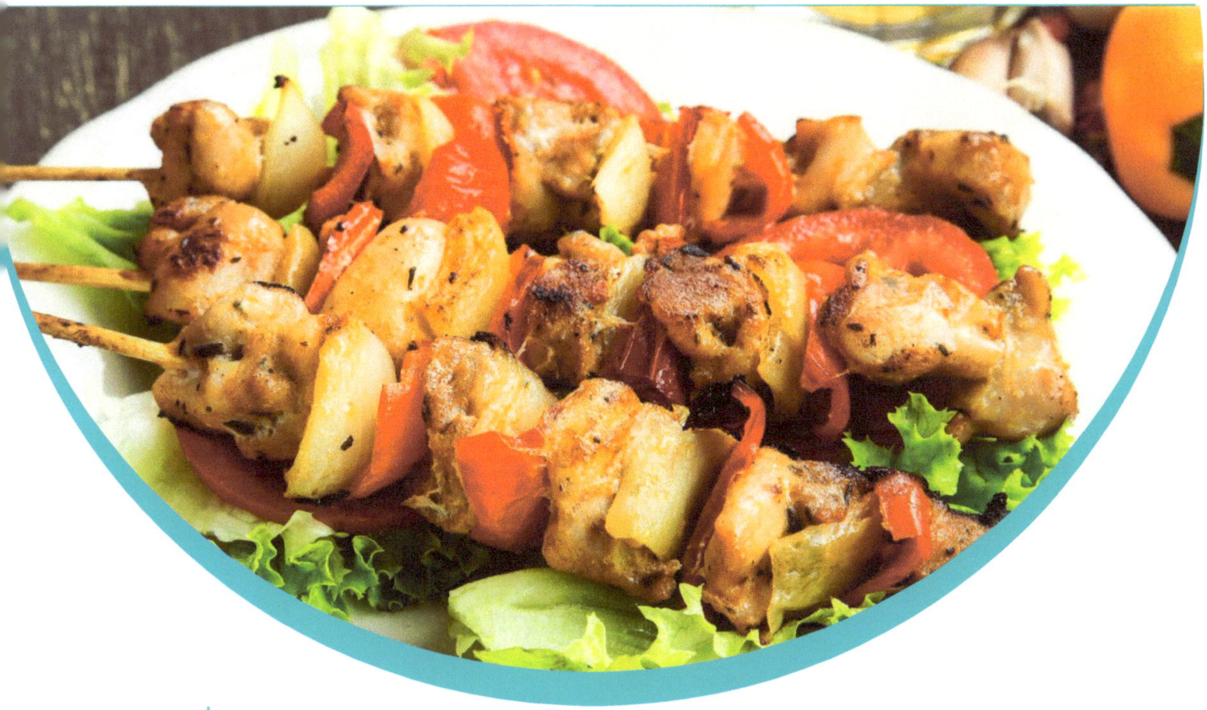

CHICKEN AND VEGETABLE SKEWERS

Ingredients

Total Time:
15 Mins

Serving:
4

1 lb boneless, skinless chicken breasts cut into cubes
1 zucchini, cut into rounds
1 red onion
1 red bell pepper, cut into squares
1 yellow bell pepper, cut into squares
2 tablespoons olive oil

1 tablespoon low-sodium soy sauce
1 teaspoon garlic powder
Salt and pepper to taste

Directions

1. Preheat the grill to medium-high heat.
2. Whisk together olive oil, soy sauce, garlic powder, salt, and pepper in a large bowl.
3. Add chicken and vegetables to the bowl and toss to coat evenly.
4. Thread chicken and vegetables onto skewers.
5. Grill skewers for 10-12 minutes, turning occasionally, until chicken is cooked through and vegetables are tender.

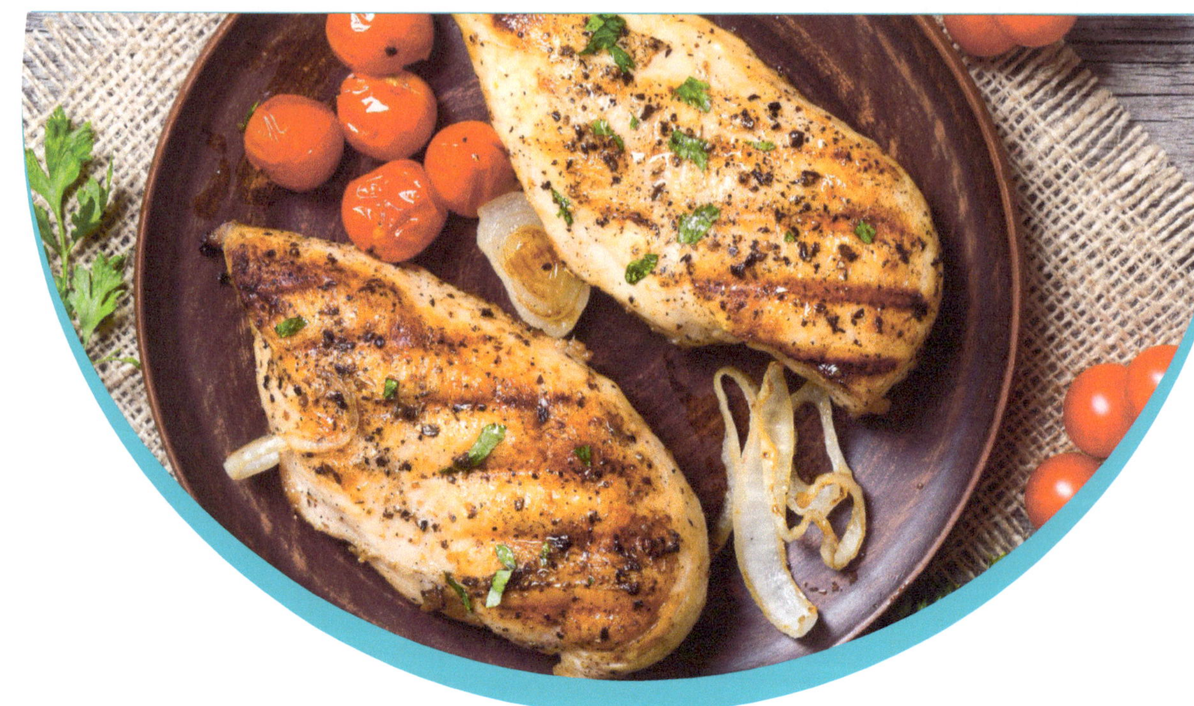

MEDITERRANEAN GRILLED CHICKEN

**Total Time:
20 Mins**

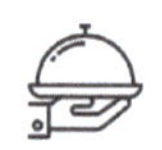

**Serving:
2**

Ingredients

4 boneless, skinless chicken breasts
2 tablespoons olive oil
2 garlic cloves, minced
2 teaspoons dried oregano
1 teaspoon dried basil
1/2 teaspoon dried thyme
Salt and pepper to taste

Directions

1. Preheat the grill to medium-high heat.
2. Whisk together olive oil, garlic, oregano, basil, thyme, salt, and pepper in a small bowl.
3. Brush the mixture over both sides of the chicken breasts.
4. Grill chicken for 6-7 minutes per side until chicken is cooked through.

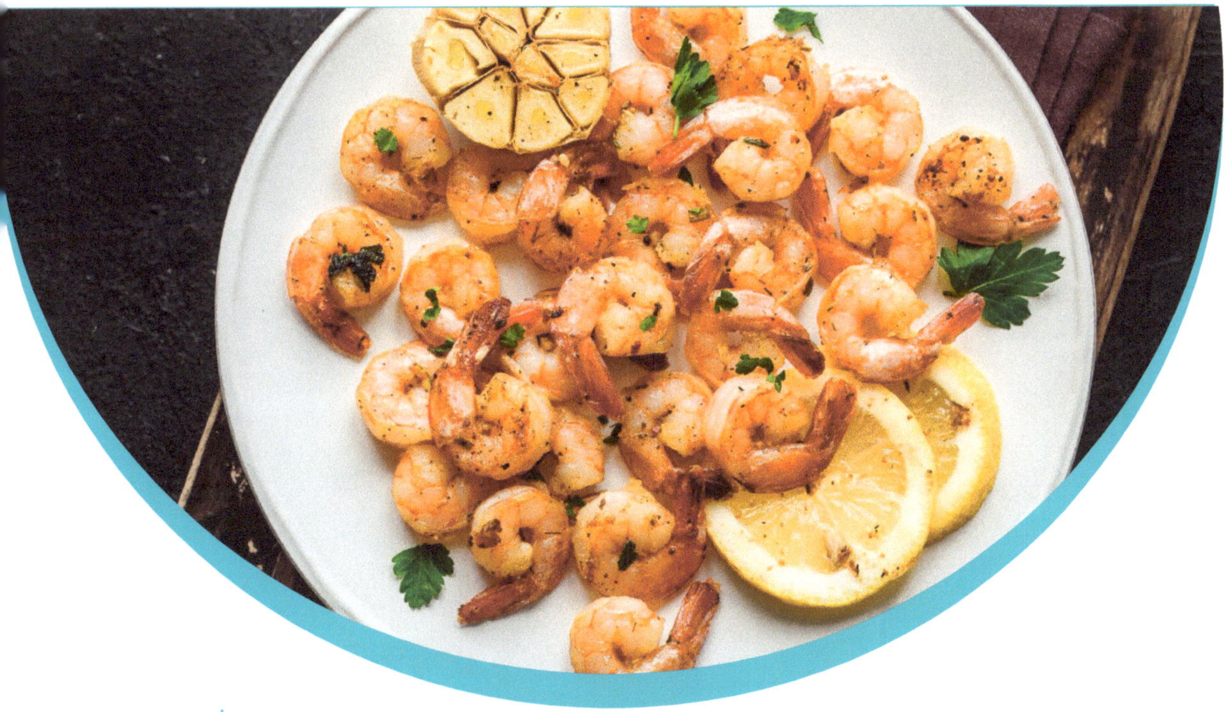

LEMON GARLIC SHRIMP

Ingredients

Total Time:
10 Mins

Serving:
4

1 lb large shrimp, peeled and
deveined
2 tablespoons olive oil
2 garlic cloves, minced
1 lemon, juiced
1 tablespoon chopped fresh parsley
Salt and pepper to taste

Directions

1. In a large skillet, heat olive oil over medium-high heat.
2. Add garlic and cook for 1-2 minutes, until fragrant.
3. Add shrimp and cook for 2-3 minutes per side until pink and cooked through.
4. Add lemon juice and parsley to the skillet and stir to combine.
5. Season with salt and pepper to taste.

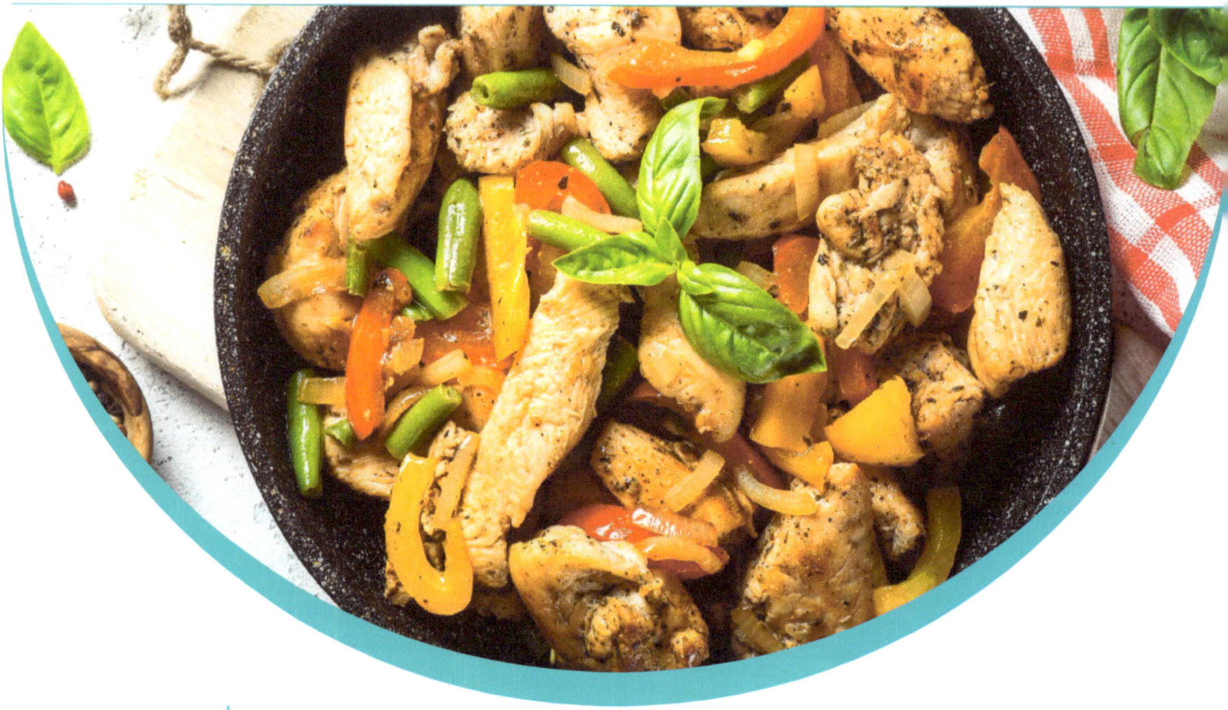

TOMATO BASIL CHICKEN

Ingredients

**Total Time:
35 Mins**

**Serving:
4**

4 boneless, skinless chicken breasts
1 tablespoon olive oil
2 garlic cloves, minced
2 cups cherry tomatoes, halved
1/4 cup chopped fresh basil
Salt and pepper to taste

Directions

1. Preheat oven to 375°F.
2. In a large oven-safe skillet, heat olive oil over medium-high heat.
3. Add garlic and cook for 1-2 minutes, until fragrant.
4. Add chicken and cook for 3-4 minutes per side until browned.
5. Remove chicken from skillet and set aside.
6. Add cherry tomatoes to the skillet and cook for 2-3 minutes, until they soften.
7. Return chicken to the skillet and spoon tomato mixture over the top.
8. Bake for 15-20 minutes, until chicken is cooked through.
9. Sprinkle with chopped basil before serving.

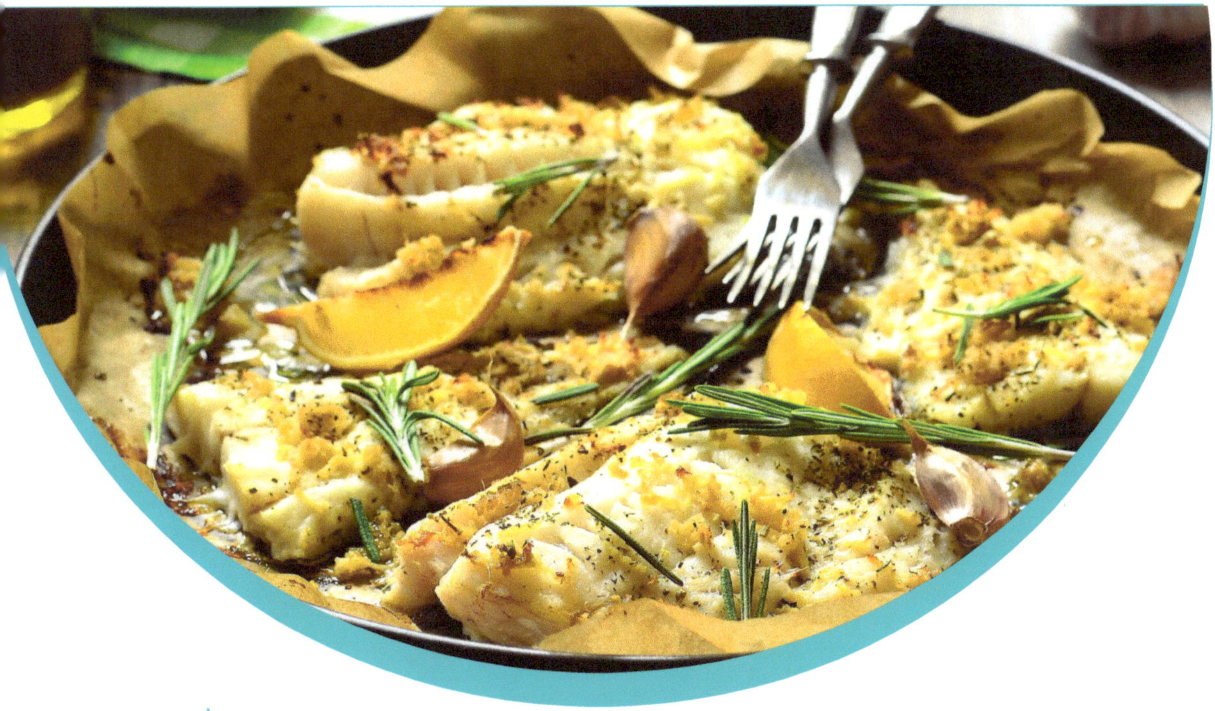

**Total Time:
25 Mins**

**Serving:
6**

LEMON HERB BAKED COD

Ingredients

4 cod fillets
2 tablespoons olive oil
1 lemon, juiced
2 garlic cloves, minced
1 teaspoon dried thyme
Salt and pepper to taste

Directions

1. Preheat oven to 375°F.
2. Whisk together olive oil, lemon juice, garlic, thyme, salt, and pepper in a small bowl.
3. Place cod fillets on a baking sheet lined with parchment paper.
4. Brush the lemon-herb mixture over the top of the cod.
5. Bake for 12-15 minutes, until cod is cooked through.

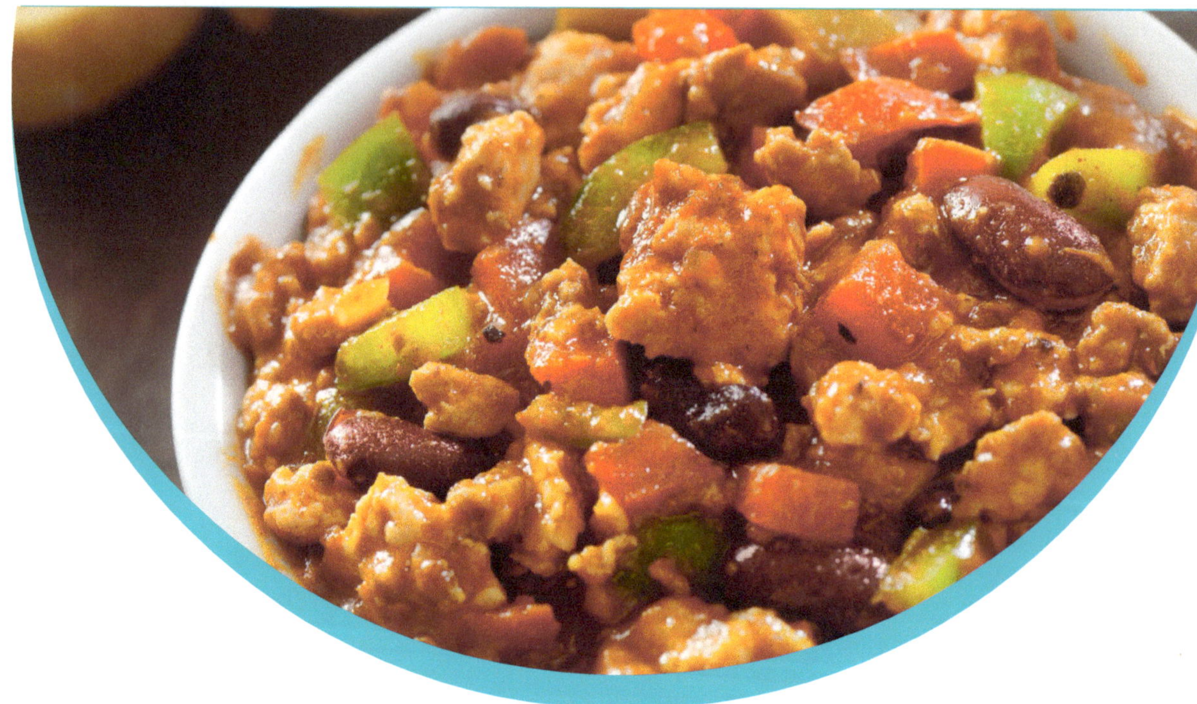

TURKEY AND VEGETABLE CHILI

Ingredients

**Total Time:
35 Mins**

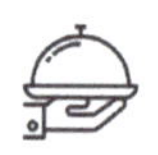

**Serving:
4**

1 lb ground turkey
1 tablespoon olive oil
1 onion, chopped
2 garlic cloves, minced
1 green bell pepper, chopped
1 red bell pepper, chopped
2 zucchinis, chopped
1 can (15 oz) low-sodium kidney

beans, drained and rinsed
1 can (14.5 oz) diced tomatoes, undrained
1 cup low-sodium chicken broth
2 tablespoons chili powder
1 teaspoon ground cumin
Salt and pepper to taste

Directions

1. Heat olive oil over medium-high heat in a large pot or Dutch oven.
2. Add onion and garlic and cook for 1-2 minutes, until fragrant.
3. Add ground turkey and cook for 5-7 minutes, until browned.
4. Add green and red bell peppers, zucchini, kidney beans, diced tomatoes, chicken broth, chili powder, cumin, salt, and pepper.
5. Stir to combine and bring to a boil.
6. Reduce heat to low and let simmer for 20-25 minutes, until vegetables are tender and chili has thickened.

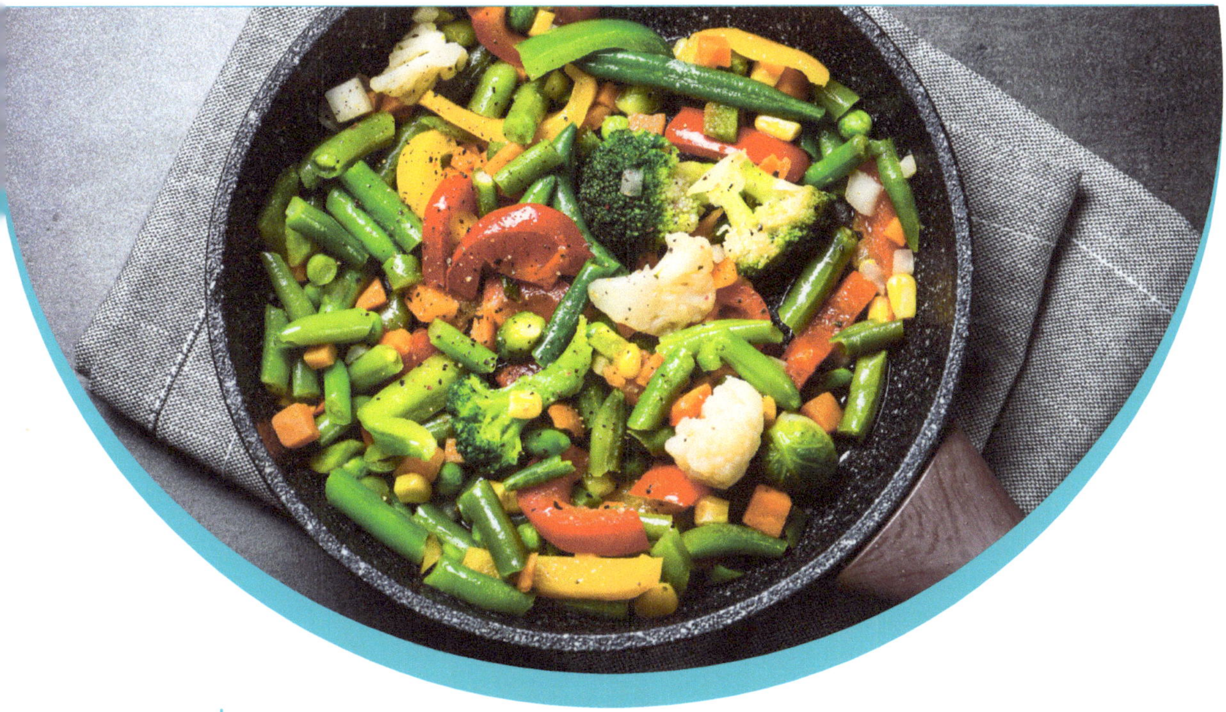

VEGETABLE STIR-FRY

Ingredients

Total Time:
15 Mins

Serving:
2

1 tablespoon olive oil
1 onion, chopped
2 garlic cloves, minced
2 cups mixed vegetables (such as broccoli, carrots, snow peas, and bell peppers), chopped
1 tablespoon low-sodium soy sauce
Salt and pepper to taste

Directions

1. In a large skillet, heat olive oil over medium-high heat.
2. Add onion and garlic and cook for 1-2 minutes, until fragrant.
3. Add mixed vegetables and cook for 5-7 minutes, until vegetables are tender.
4. Stir in low-sodium soy sauce and season with salt and pepper to taste.
5. Serve over cooked brown rice or quinoa, if desired.

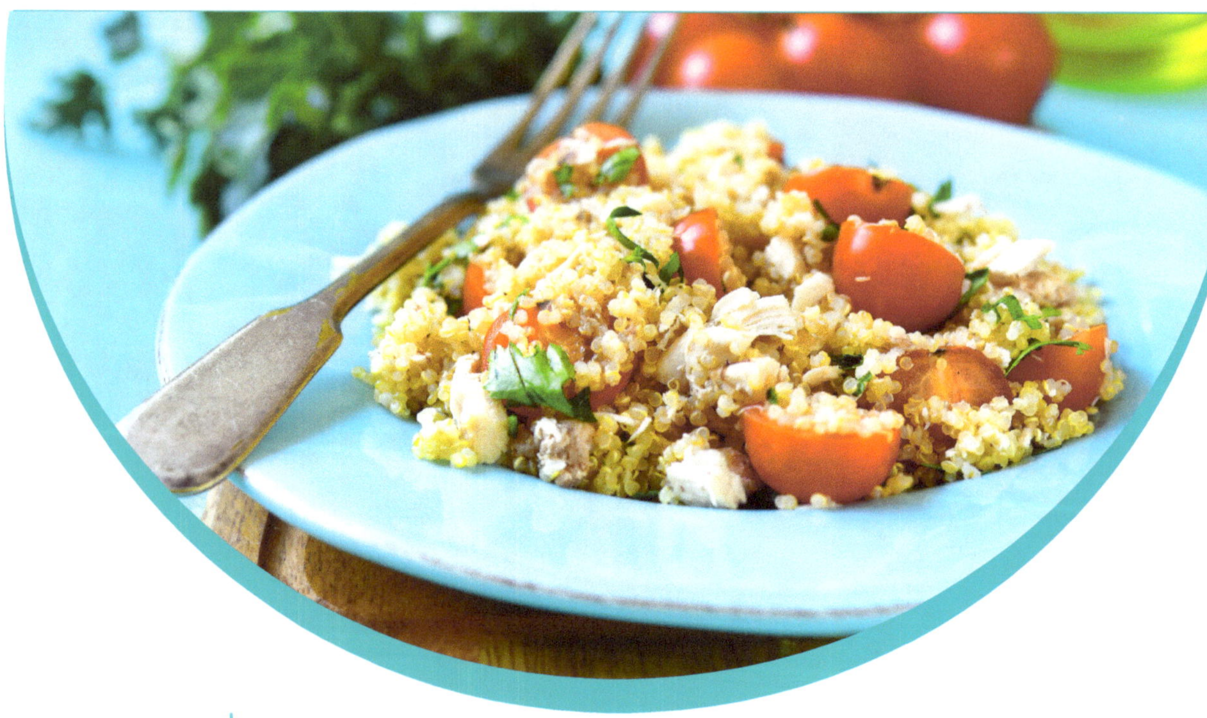

QUINOA SALAD WITH CHERRY

Total Time:
25 Mins

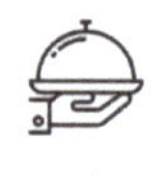

Serving:
4

Ingredients

1 cup quinoa, rinsed
2 cups water
2 grilled chicken breasts, sliced
1 pint cherry tomatoes, halved
1 avocado, diced
1/4 cup red onion, diced
1/4 cup cilantro, chopped
Juice of 1 lime

2 tbsp. olive oil
Salt and pepper, to taste

Directions

1. In a medium saucepan, bring quinoa and water to a boil.
2. Reduce heat to low and simmer for 15-20 minutes or until the quinoa is cooked.
3. Combine cooked quinoa, sliced chicken, cherry tomatoes, avocado, red onion, and cilantro
4. in a large bowl.
5. Whisk together lime juice, olive oil, salt, and pepper in a small bowl.
6. Pour the dressing over the quinoa salad and toss to combine.
7. Serve chilled.

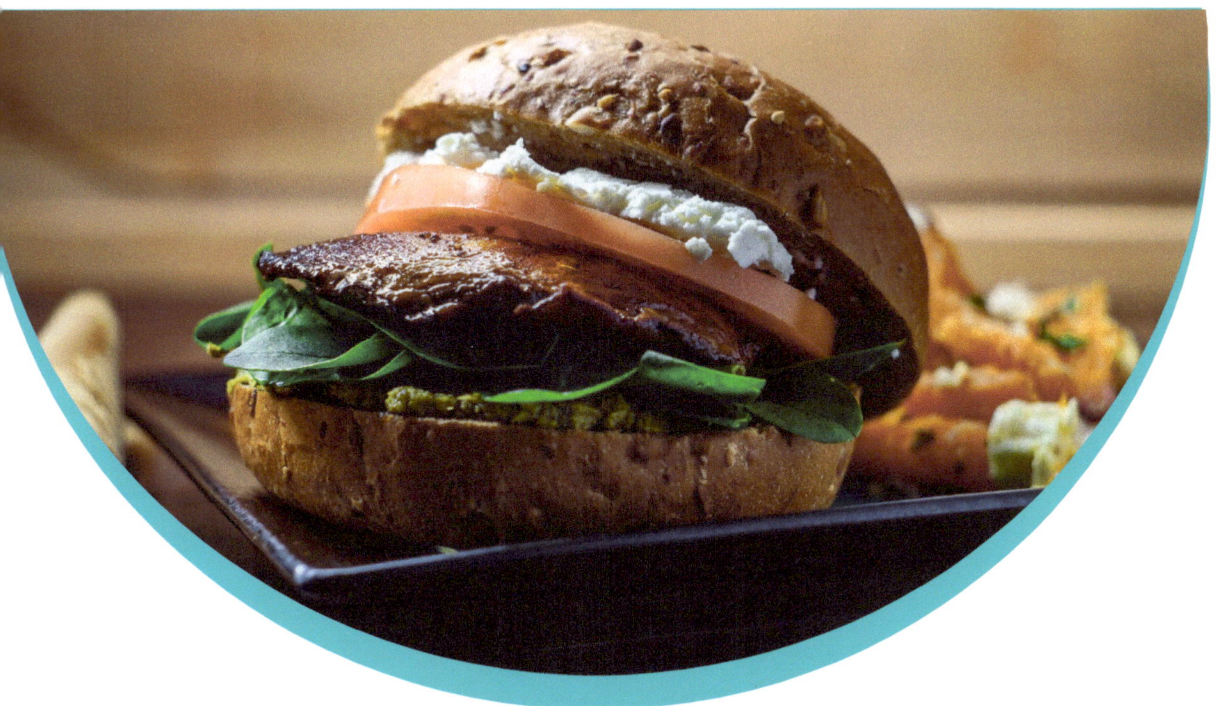

GRILLED PORTOBELLO MUSHROOM BURGER

**Total Time:
40 Mins**

**Serving:
4**

Ingredients

4 portobello mushroom caps
1 tbsp. olive oil
2 garlic cloves, minced
Salt and pepper, to taste
4 whole wheat burger buns
1 sweet potato, cut into wedges
1 tbsp. coconut oil

Directions

1. Preheat the grill to medium-high heat. Combine olive oil, minced garlic, salt, and pepper in a small bowl.
2. Brush the portobello mushroom caps with the garlic and olive oil mixture.
3. Grill the mushroom caps for 5-7 minutes per side or until they are tender and charred.
4. While the mushrooms are cooking, preheat the oven to 400°F.
5. Toss sweet potato wedges with coconut oil, salt, and pepper.
6. Spread the sweet potato wedges on a baking sheet and roast for 20-25 minutes or until tender.
7. Serve the grilled mushroom caps on whole wheat burger buns with roasted sweet potato wedges.

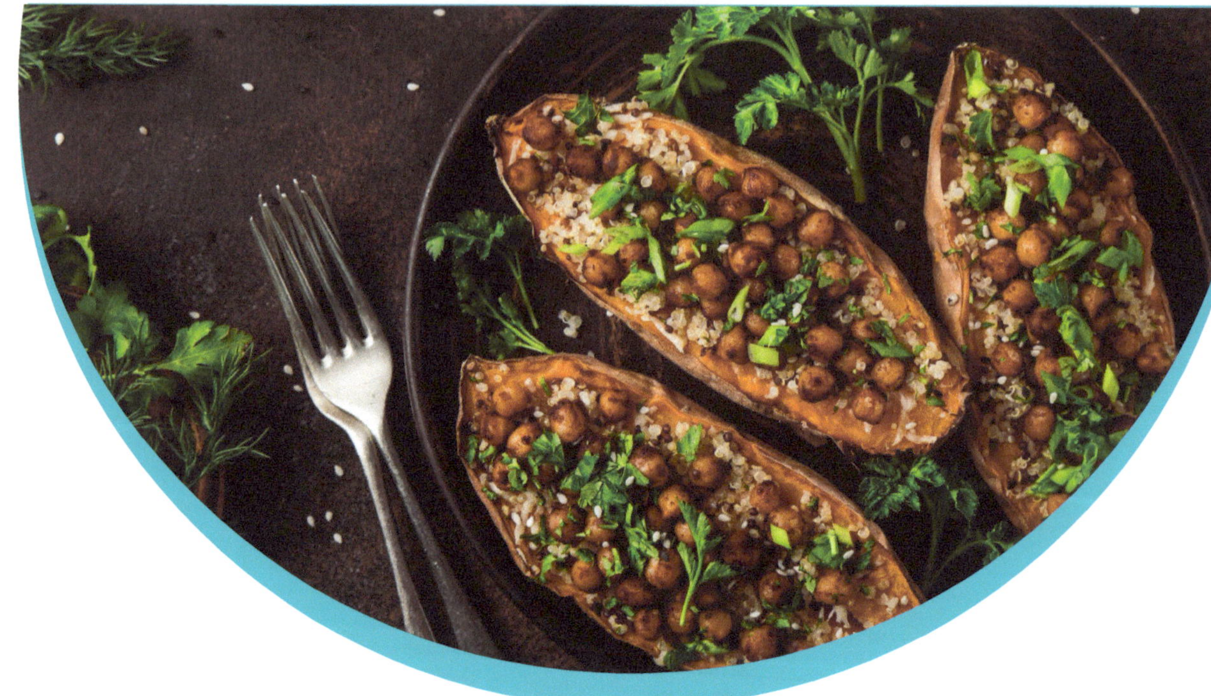

MEDITERRANEAN STUFFED SWEET POTATOES

Ingredients

**Total Time:
1 hour 10
mins**

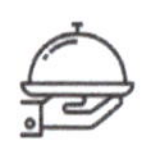

**Serving:
2**

2 medium sweet potatoes
1/2 cup canned chickpeas, rinsed
and drained
1/2 cup diced tomatoes
1/4 cup diced red onion
1/4 cup crumbled feta cheese
2 tbsp chopped fresh parsley
2 tbsp olive oil

1 tbsp red wine vinegar
Salt and pepper, to taste

Directions

1. Preheat oven to 400°F.
2. Pierce sweet potatoes with a fork and bake for 45-50 minutes or until tender.
3. Mix a bowl of chickpeas, tomatoes, red onion, feta cheese, parsley, olive oil, vinegar, salt, and pepper.
4. Once sweet potatoes are cooked, slice them in half lengthwise and scoop some of the flesh.
5. Stuff the chickpea mixture into the sweet potatoes.
6. Bake for an additional 10 minutes.

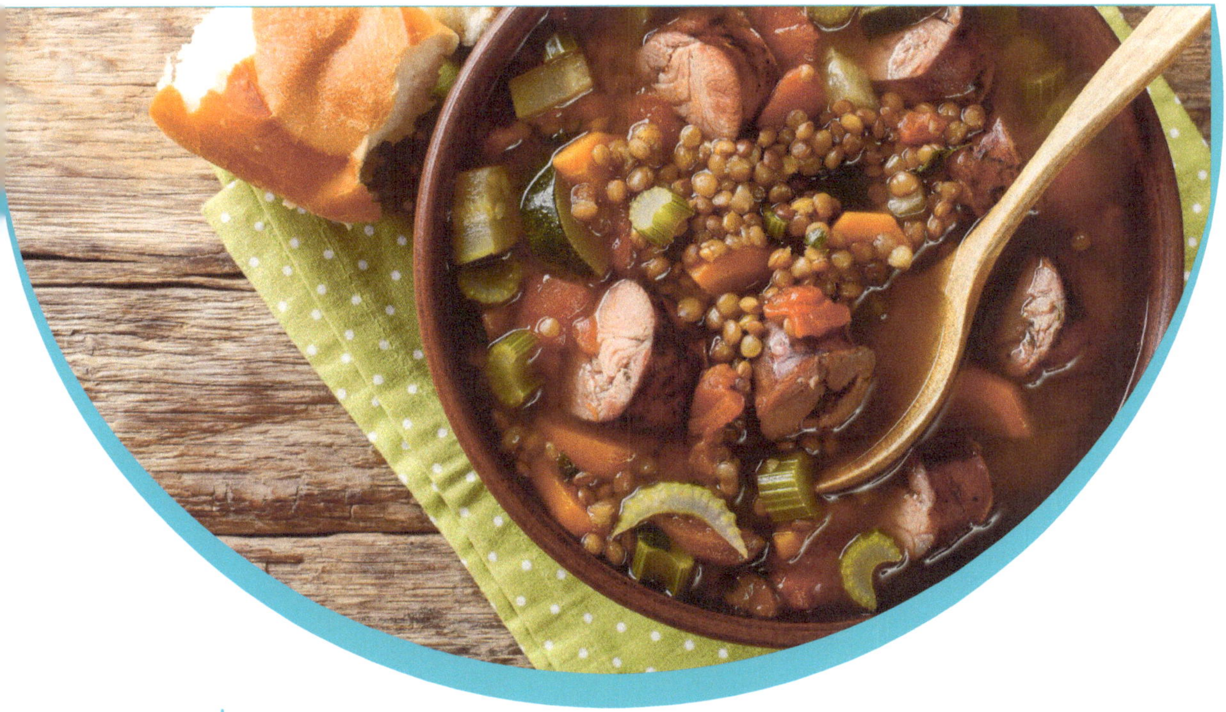

ZUCCHINI AND LENTIL SOUP

Total Time:
40 Mins

Serving:
4

Ingredients

1 tbsp. olive oil
1 onion, diced
2 garlic cloves, minced
2 zucchinis, diced
1 cup dried green lentils, rinsed
4 cups low-sodium vegetable broth
1 bay leaf
1 tsp. dried thyme

Salt and pepper, to taste
Whole grain bread for serving

Directions

1. In a large pot, heat olive oil over medium heat.
2. Add diced onion and minced garlic and cook until the onion is soft and translucent.
3. Add chopped zucchini and cook for another 2-3 minutes.
4. Add rinsed green lentils, vegetable broth, bay leaf, dried thyme, salt, and pepper.
5. Bring the soup to a boil, then reduce the heat and let it simmer for 25-30 minutes or until the lentils are tender.
6. Remove the bay leaf and serve the soup with a slice of whole grain bread.

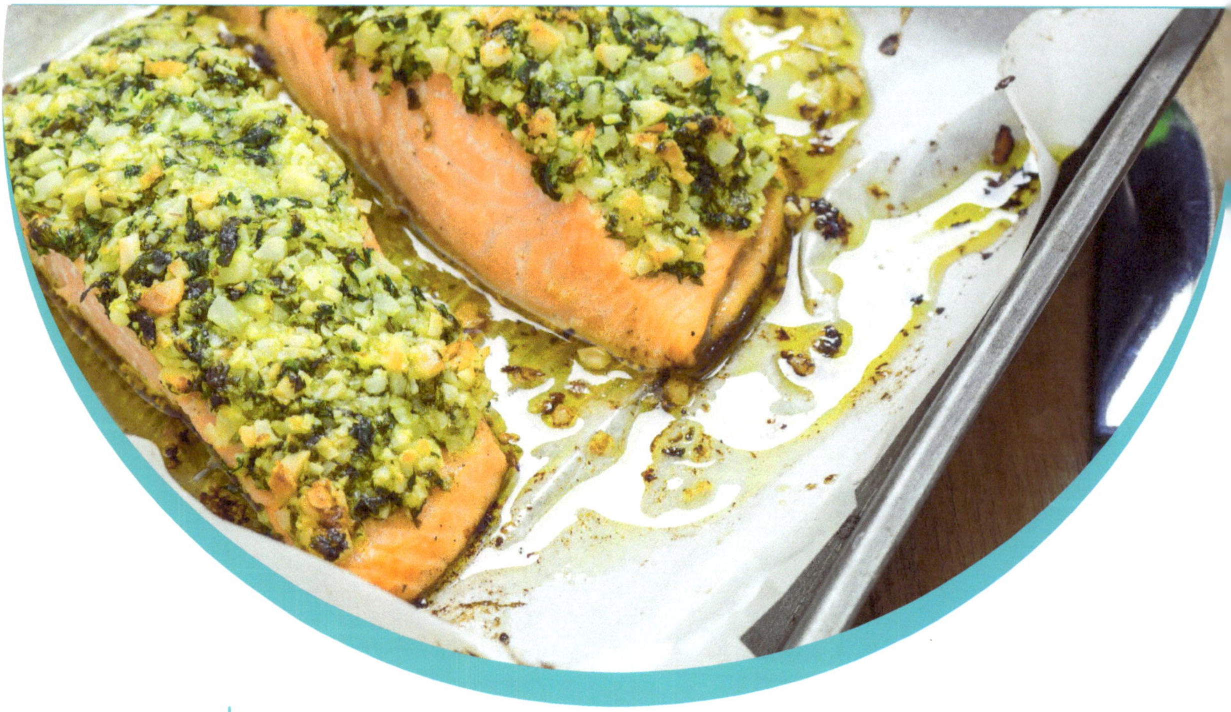

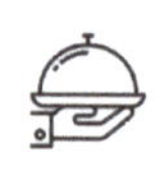

BAKED SALMON WITH HERB CRUST

Ingredients

**Total Time:
50 Mins**

**Serving:
6**

4 salmon fillets
1/2 cup panko breadcrumbs
2 tbsp fresh parsley, chopped
2 tbsp fresh dill, chopped
2 tbsp fresh chives, chopped
1 lemon, zested
2 tbsp olive oil
Salt and pepper, to taste

Directions

1. Preheat oven to 375°F.
2. Combine breadcrumbs, parsley, dill, chives, lemon zest, olive oil, salt, and pepper in a small bowl.
3. Mix until well combined.
4. Place salmon fillets on a baking sheet and season with salt and pepper.
5. Spread the herb mixture evenly over the top of each fillet.
6. Bake for 12-15 minutes or until salmon is cooked through.
7. Spread the Brussels sprouts on a baking sheet and roast for 20-25 minutes until tender and browned. Drizzle the roasted Brussels sprouts with balsamic vinegar.
8. Serve the grilled shrimp skewers with quinoa and roasted Brussels sprouts.

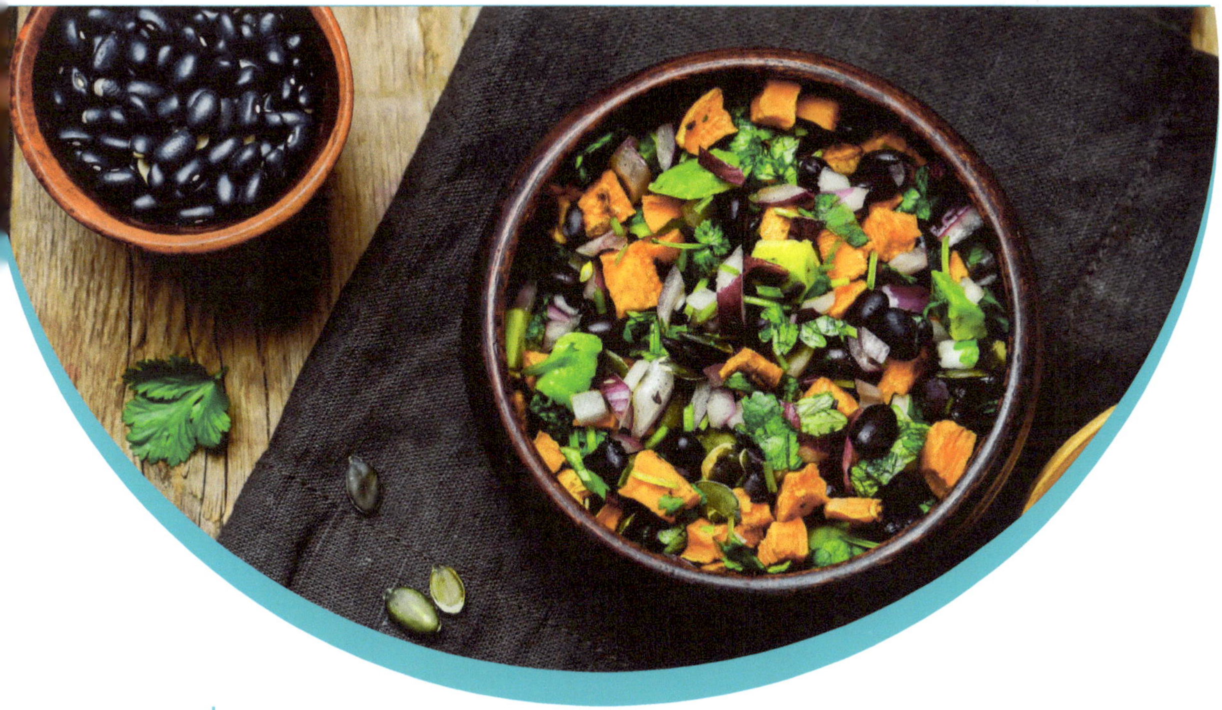

SWEET POTATO AND BLACK BEAN CHILI

Total Time:
40 Mins

Serving:
4

Ingredients

1 tbsp. olive oil
1 onion, diced
2 garlic cloves, minced
1 sweet potato, peeled and diced
1 can (15 oz.) black beans, rinsed
and drained
1 can (15 oz.) diced tomatoes
1 tbsp. chili powder

1 tsp. ground cumin
Salt and pepper, to taste
2 cups cooked brown rice

Directions

1. In a large pot, heat olive oil over medium heat.
2. Add diced onion and minced garlic and cook until the onion is soft and translucent.
3. Add diced sweet potato and cook for another 5-7 minutes.
4. Add rinsed black beans, diced tomatoes (with their juices), chili powder, ground cumin, salt, and pepper.
5. Bring the chili to a boil, then reduce heat and let it simmer for 20-25 minutes or until the sweet potato is tender.
6. Serve the sweet potato and black bean chili with a side of cooked brown rice.

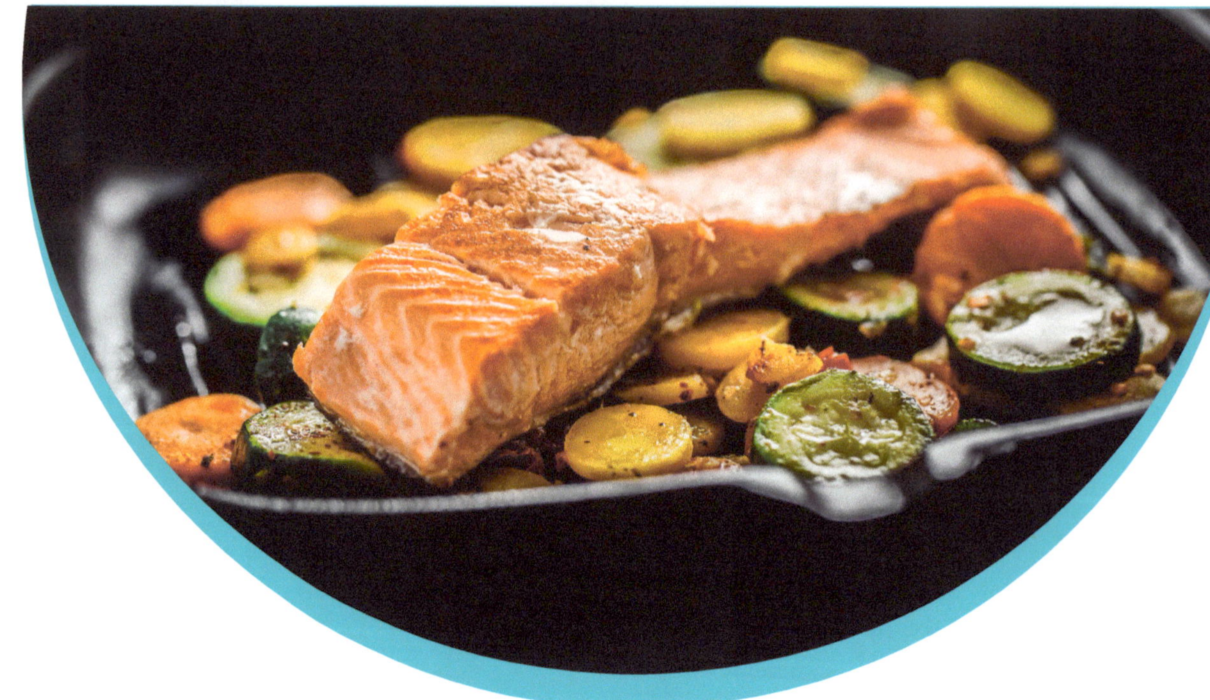

BAKED SALMON WITH ROASTED VEGETABLES

**Total Time:
45 Mins**

**Serving:
4**

Ingredients

4 salmon fillets
1 tbsp. olive oil
1 lemon, sliced
Salt and pepper, to taste
1 lb. asparagus, trimmed
1 lb. carrots, peeled and cut into
sticks
1 red onion, cut into wedges

Directions

1. Preheat oven to 400°F.
2. Place the salmon fillets on a baking sheet lined with parchment paper.
3. Drizzle olive oil over the salmon fillets and season with salt and pepper.
4. Arrange lemon slices on top of the salmon fillets.
5. In a separate bowl, toss asparagus, carrots, and red onion with olive oil, salt, and pepper.
6. Spread the vegetables on a separate baking sheet and roast for 20-25 minutes until tender and browned.
7. Bake the salmon fillets for 10-12 minutes or until cooked through.
8. Serve the baked salmon with a side of roasted vegetables.

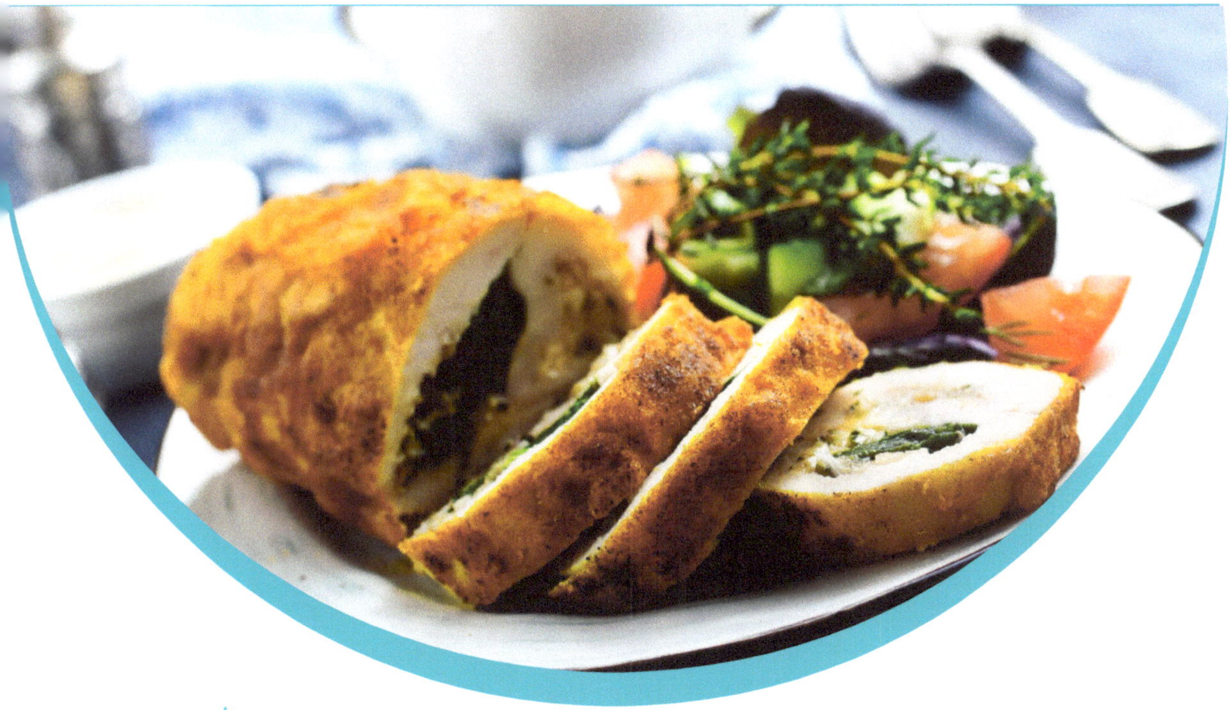

SPINACH AND FETA STUFFED CHICKEN BREAST

Ingredients

Total Time:
55 Mins

Serving:
4

4 boneless, skinless chicken breasts
1 tbsp. olive oil
2 garlic cloves, minced
4 cups spinach leaves
1/2 cup crumbled feta cheese
Salt and pepper, to taste
1 cup quinoa, rinsed
2 cups water

Directions

1. Preheat oven to 375°F. In a large skillet, heat olive oil over medium heat.
2. Add minced garlic and cook until fragrant, about 1 minute. Add spinach leaves and cook until wilted, about 2-3 minutes.
3. Remove the skillet from heat and stir in crumbled feta cheese.
4. Cut a pocket into each chicken breast and stuff with the spinach and feta mixture Season the chicken breasts with salt and pepper.
5. Place the stuffed chicken breasts on a baking sheet lined with parchment paper.
6. Bake for 25-30 minutes until the chicken is cooked through.
7. In a medium saucepan, bring quinoa and water to a boil.
8. Reduce heat to low and simmer for 15-20 minutes until the quinoa is cooked.
9. Serve the spinach, and feta stuffed chicken breast with a side of cooked quinoa.

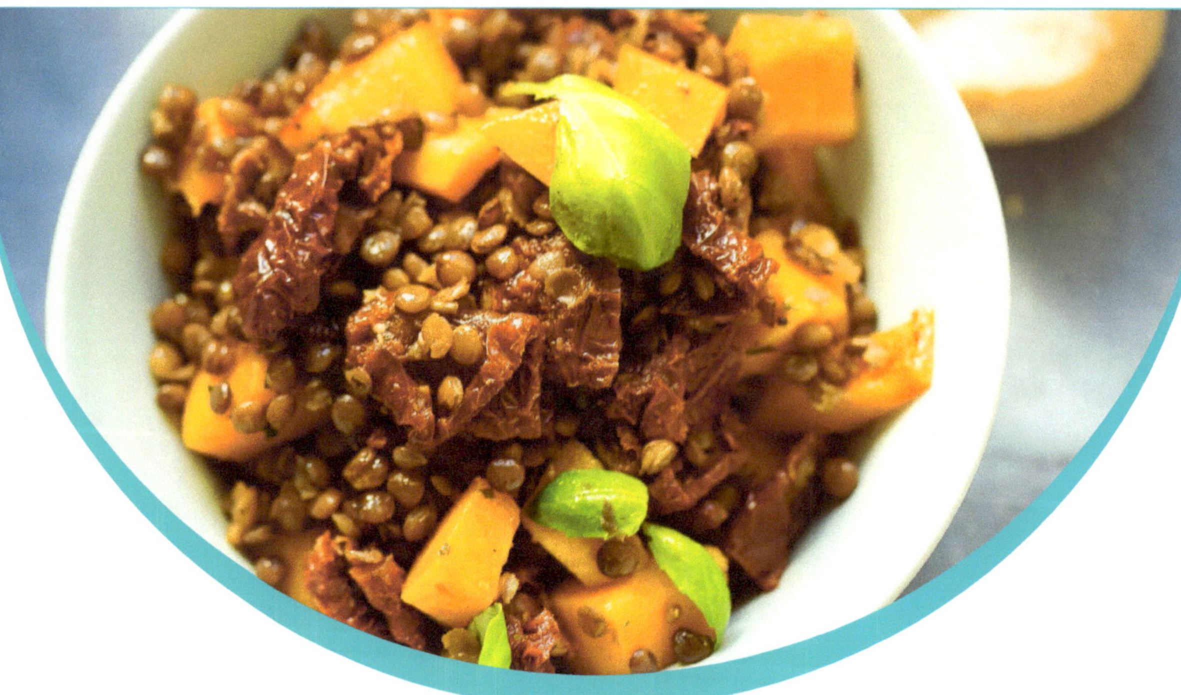

LENTIL AND VEGETABLE STIR-FRY

Ingredients

**Total Time:
40 Mins**

**Serving:
4**

1 cup dried green lentils, rinsed
2 cups water
1 tbsp. olive oil
1 onion, diced
2 garlic cloves, minced
2 cups mixed vegetables (e.g.,
broccoli, bell peppers, carrots,
mushrooms)

2 tbsp. low-sodium soy sauce
Salt and pepper, to taste
Brown rice, for serving

Directions

1. In a medium saucepan, bring lentils and water to a boil.
2. Reduce heat to low and simmer for 20-25 minutes or until the lentils are tender.
3. Drain any excess water from the lentils and set them aside.
4. In a large skillet, heat olive oil over medium heat.
5. Add diced onion and minced garlic and cook until the onion is soft and translucent.
6. Add mixed vegetables and stir-fry for 5-7 minutes until tender but slightly crisp.
7. Add the cooked lentils to the skillet and stir to combine.
8. Pour low-sodium soy sauce over the lentil and vegetable mixture and stir to coat.
9. Season with salt and pepper to taste.
10. Serve the lentil and vegetable stir-fry with a side of cooked brown rice.

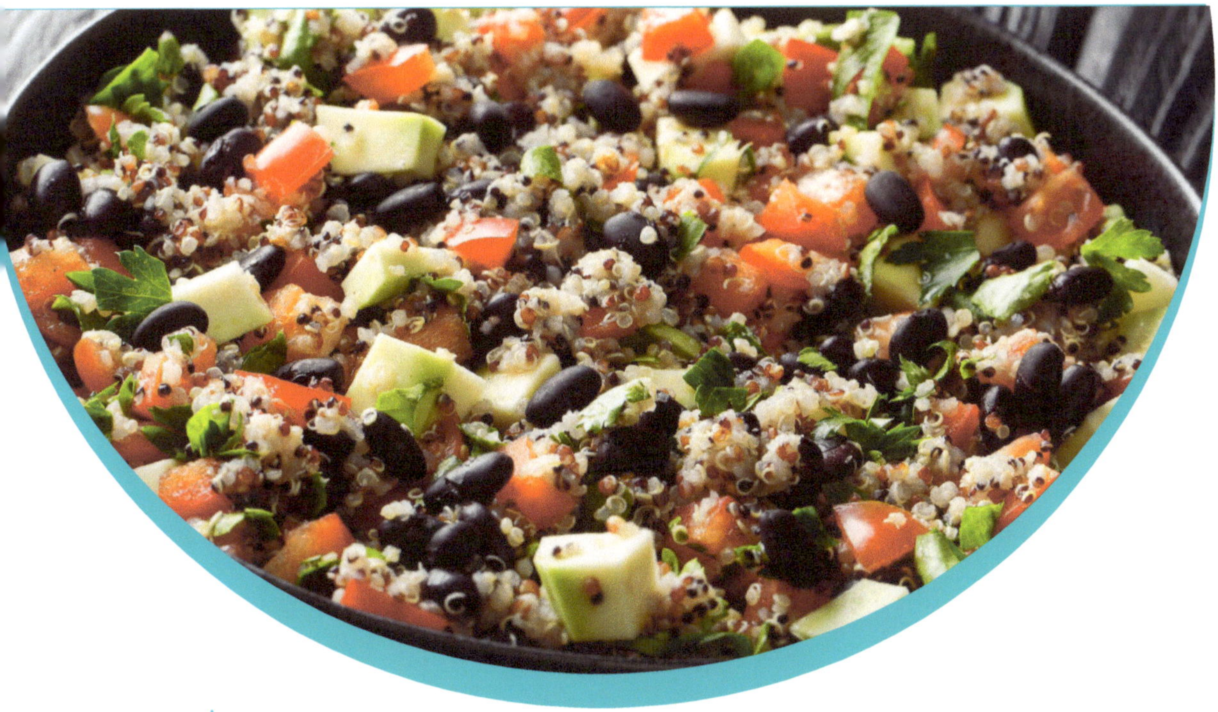

QUINOA AND BLACK BEAN SALAD

**Total Time:
25 Mins**

**Serving:
2**

Ingredients

1 cup quinoa, rinsed
2 cups water
1 can low-sodium black beans,
drained and rinsed
1 red bell pepper, diced
1/2 red onion, diced
1/4 cup chopped cilantro
1 lime, juiced

1 tbsp. olive oil
Salt and pepper, to taste

Directions

1. In a medium saucepan, bring quinoa and water to a boil.
2. Reduce heat to low and simmer for 15-20 minutes until the quinoa is cooked.
3. Combine cooked quinoa, black beans, diced red bell pepper, red onion, and chopped cilantro in a large bowl.
4. In a separate small bowl, whisk together lime juice and olive oil.
5. Pour the lime and olive oil dressing over the quinoa and black bean salad and stir to combine.
6. Season with salt and pepper to taste.
7. Serve the quinoa and black bean salad chilled.

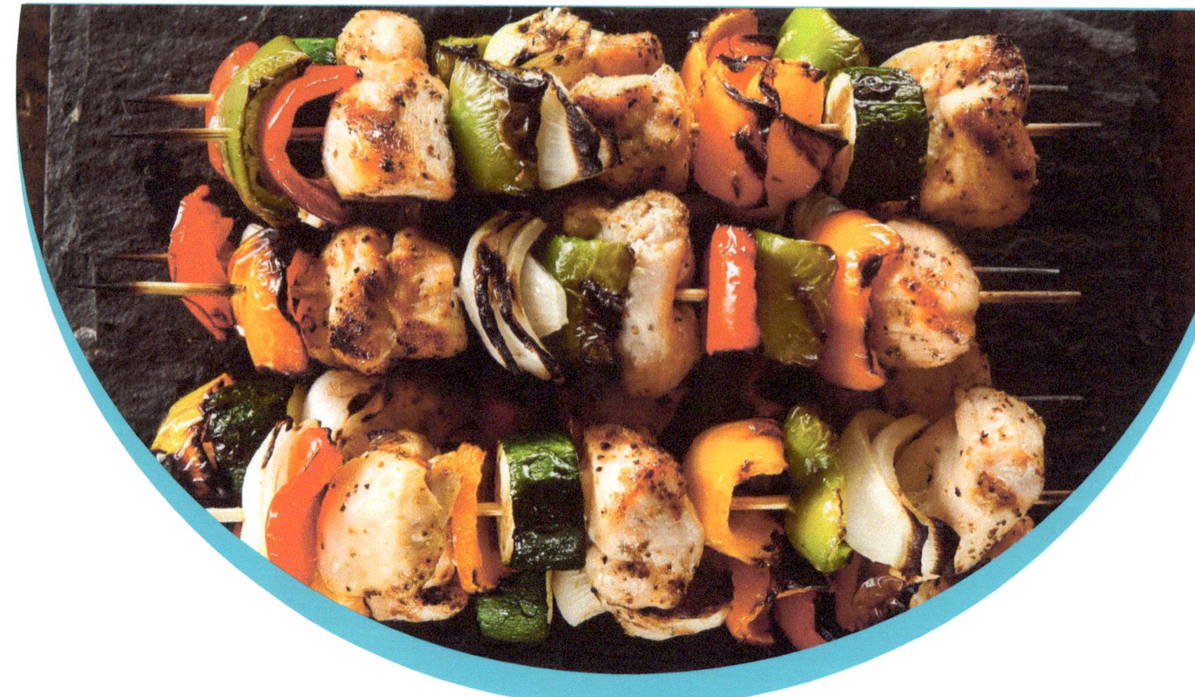

GRILLED CHICKEN AND VEGETABLE KABOBS

**Total Time:
20 Mins**

**Serving:
2**

Ingredients

4 boneless, skinless chicken breasts cut into cubes

1 red bell pepper, cut into chunks

1 yellow bell pepper, cut into chunks

1 zucchini, sliced

1 red onion, cut into chunks

1 tbsp. olive oil

Salt and pepper, to taste

Directions

1. Preheat the grill to medium-high heat.
2. Thread chicken cubes, red bell pepper chunks, yellow bell pepper chunks, zucchini slices, and red onion chunks onto skewers.
3. Drizzle olive oil over the kabobs and season with salt and pepper.
4. Grill the kabobs for 10-12 minutes or until the chicken is cooked through and the vegetables are tender.
5. Serve the grilled chicken and vegetable kabobs with a side of brown rice.

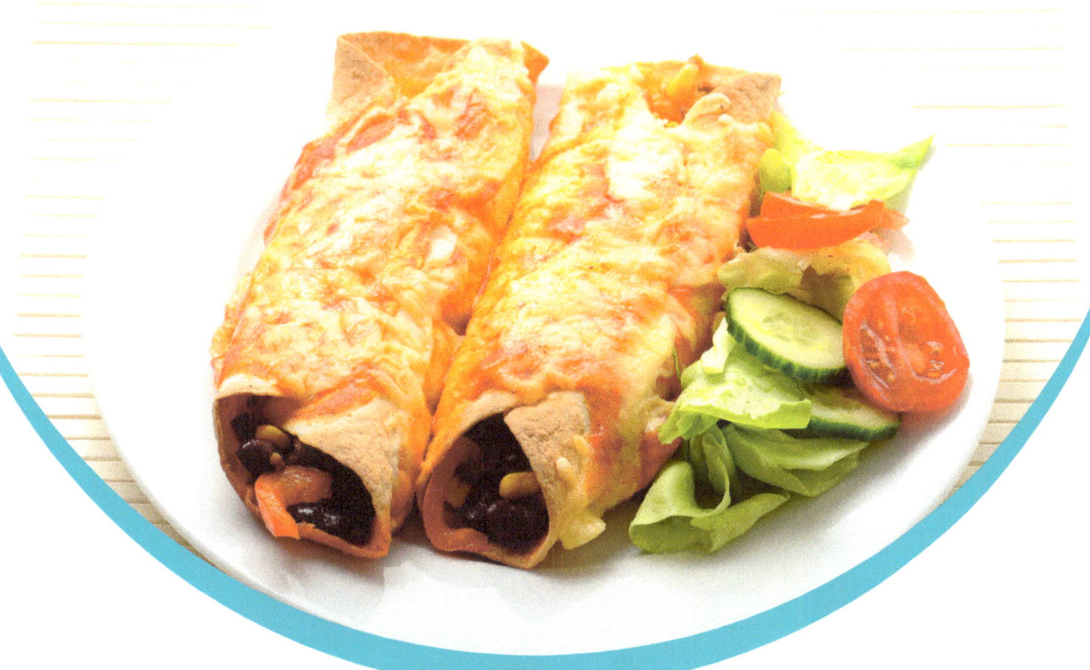

SWEET POTATO AND BLACK BEAN ENCHILADAS

Total Time:
25 Mins

Serving:
6

Ingredients

2 sweet potatoes, peeled and cubed
1 can low-sodium black beans, drained and rinsed
1 onion, diced
2 garlic cloves, minced
1 tbsp. chili powder
1 tsp. ground cumin

1 tsp. paprika
Salt and pepper, to taste
8 whole wheat tortillas
1 cup shredded cheddar cheese
Cilantro, for serving

Directions

1. Preheat oven to 375°F (190°C).
2. In a large skillet, cook diced onion and minced garlic over medium heat until softened.
3. Add cubed sweet potatoes to the skillet and cook until tender.Add drained and rinsed black beans, chili powder, ground cumin, paprika, salt, and pepper.
4. Stir to combine and cook until heated through.Place a few spoonfuls of the sweet potato and black bean mixture onto each wheat tortilla and roll up tightly.
5. Place the enchiladas in a large baking dish and sprinkle with shredded cheddar cheese. Bake for 15-20 minutes until the cheese is melted and bubbly.
6. Serve the sweet potato and black bean enchiladas with a sprinkle of fresh cilantro.

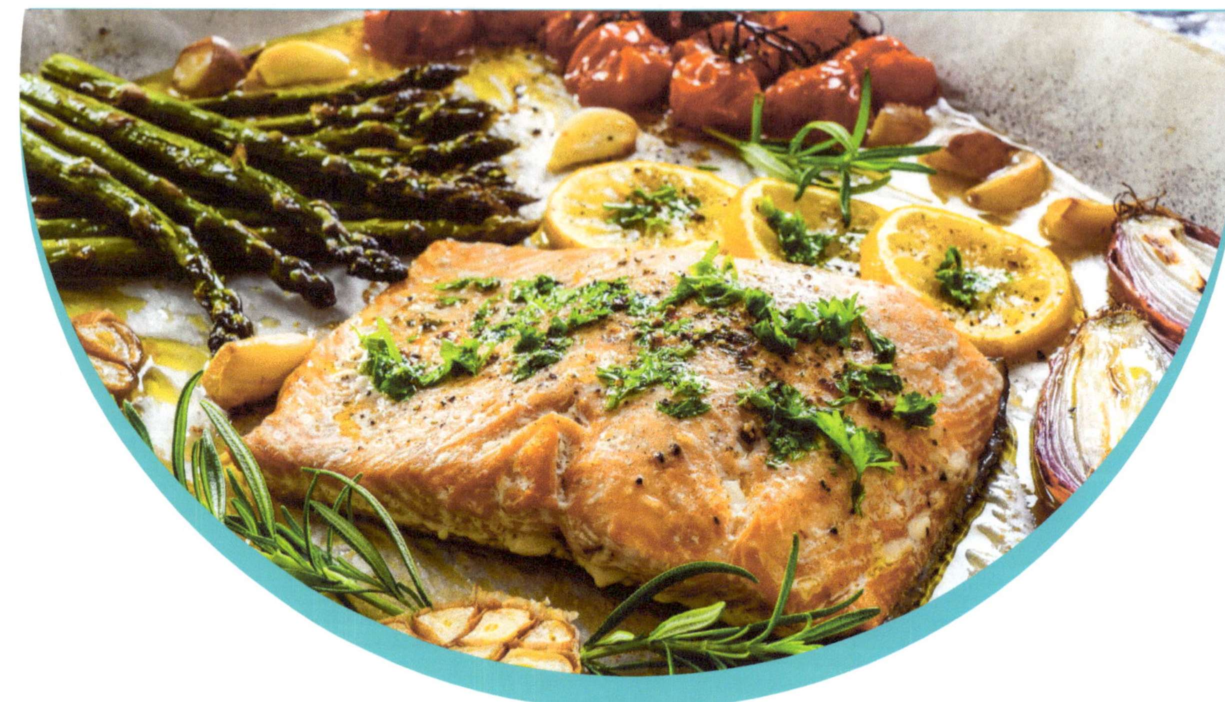

SALMON AND ASPARAGUS SHEET PAN DINNER

Total Time:
20 Mins

Serving:
2

Ingredients

4 salmon fillets
1 lb. asparagus, trimmed
1 lemon, sliced
2 tbsp. olive oil
1 tbsp. chopped fresh dill
Salt and pepper, to taste

Directions

1. Preheat oven to 425°F (220°C).
2. Arrange salmon fillets and trim asparagus on a large baking sheet.
3. Drizzle olive oil over the salmon and asparagus and season with salt and pepper.
4. Sprinkle chopped fresh dill over the top of the salmon fillets.
5. Place lemon slices on top of the salmon fillets.
6. Bake for 12-15 minutes until the salmon is cooked and the asparagus is tender.
7. Serve the salmon and asparagus sheet pan dinner with a side of cooked brown rice.

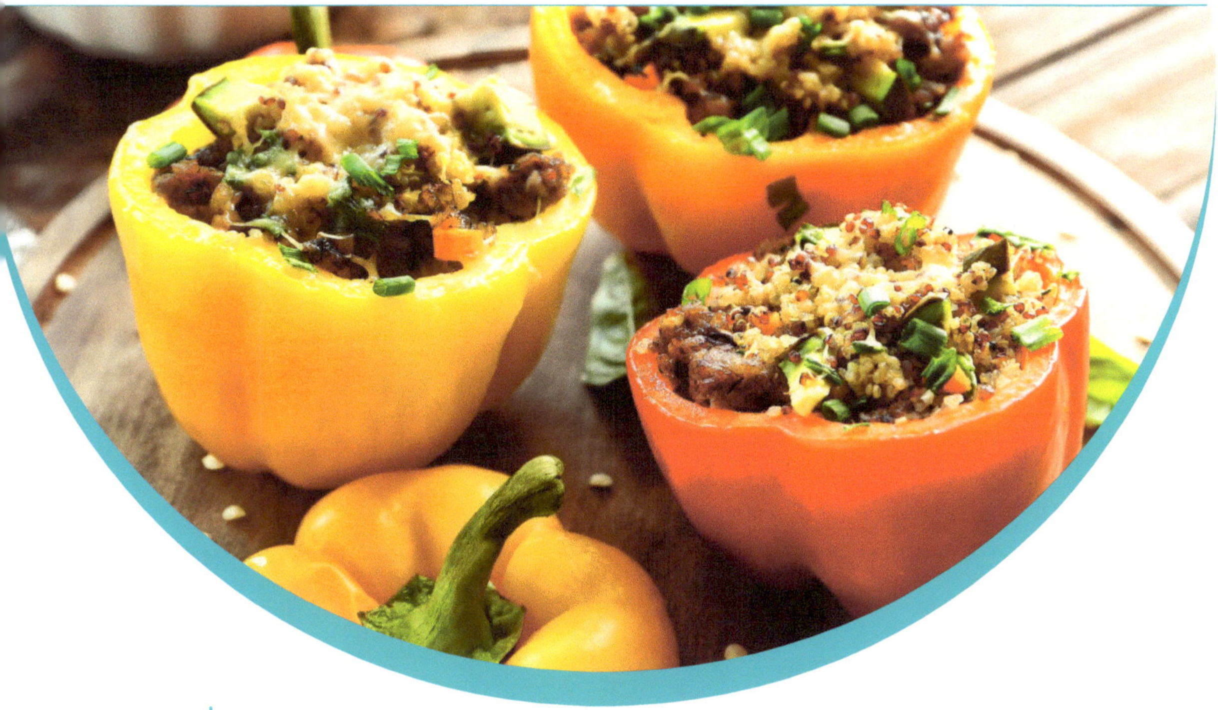

QUINOA AND VEGETABLE STUFFED BELL PEPPERS

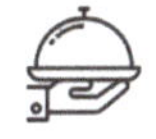

**Total Time:
60 Mins**

**Serving:
2**

Ingredients

4 bell peppers, tops removed and seeded
1 cup quinoa, rinsed
2 cups water
1 onion, diced
2 garlic cloves, minced
1 zucchini, diced
1 yellow squash, diced

1 can low-sodium diced tomatoes
1 tsp. dried oregano
Salt and pepper, to taste

Directions

1. Preheat oven to 375°F (190°C).
2. In a medium saucepan, bring quinoa and water to a boil. Reduce heat to low and simmer for 15-20 minutes until the quinoa is cooked. In a large skillet, cook diced onion and minced garlic over medium heat until softened.
3. Add chopped zucchini and yellow squash to the skillet and cook until slightly softened. Add low-sodium diced tomatoes, quinoa, dried oregano, salt, and pepper. Stir to combine and cook until heated through.
4. Stuff the quinoa and vegetable mixture into the hollowed-out bell peppers. Cover the stuffed bell peppers in a large baking dish with foil.
5. Bake for 30-35 minutes or until the bell peppers are tender. Serve the quinoa and vegetable-stuffed bell peppers hot

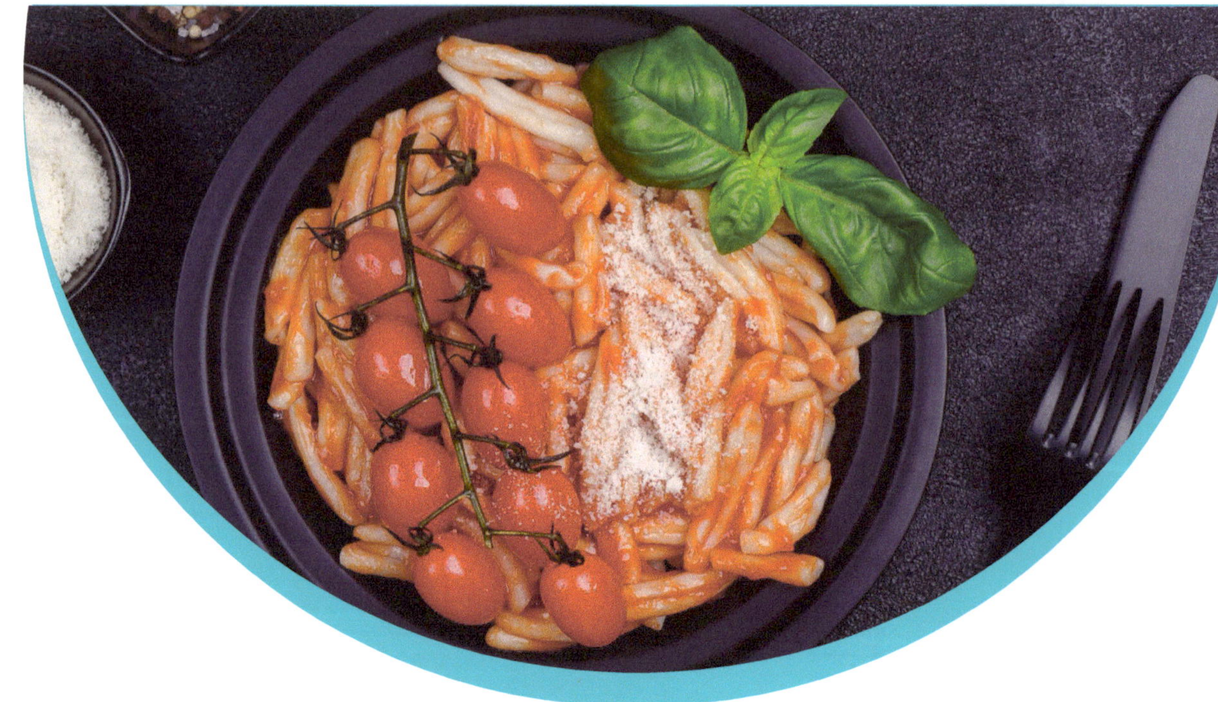

WHOLE WHEAT PASTA

**Total Time:
45 Mins**

**Serving:
2**

Ingredients

12 oz. whole wheat pasta
1 can low sodium diced tomatoes
2 garlic cloves, minced
1/4 cup chopped fresh basil
2 tbsp. olive oil
Salt and pepper, to taste
Grated parmesan cheese for
serving

Directions

1. Cook the whole wheat pasta according to the package instructions.
2. In a large skillet, heat olive oil over medium heat.
3. Add minced garlic and cook until fragrant, about 30 seconds.
4. Add low sodium diced tomatoes, chopped fresh basil, salt, and pepper to the skillet.
5. Simmer the tomato sauce for 5-10 minutes or until slightly thickened.
6. Drain the cooked pasta and add it to the skillet with the tomato sauce.
7. Toss to coat the pasta in the sauce.
8. Serve the whole wheat pasta with tomato and basil sauce topped with grated parmesan cheese.

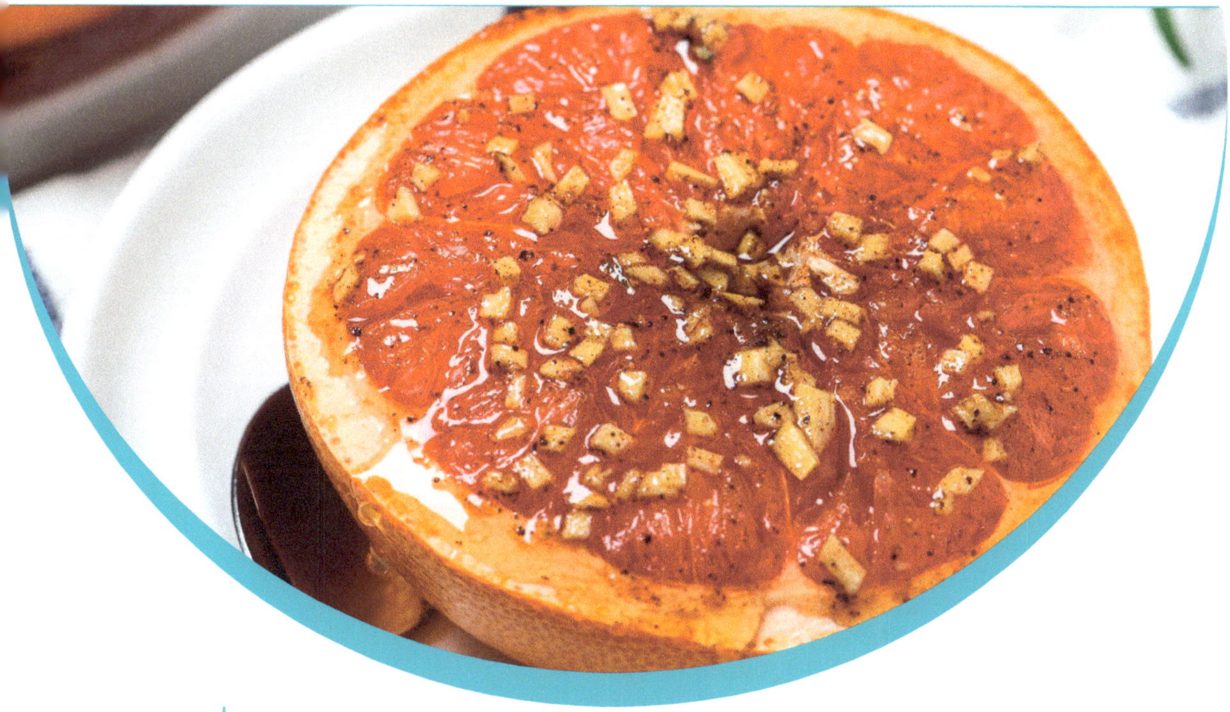

BROILED GRAPEFRUIT

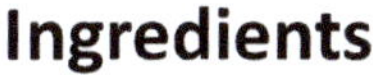

Ingredients

**Total Time:
10 Mins**

2 grapefruits, halved
2 tbsp. honey
1 tsp. Ground cinnamon

**Serving:
4**

Directions

1. Preheat the broiler.
2. Slice a thin layer off the bottom of each grapefruit half to create a flat surface.
3. Use a paring knife to loosen the grapefruit segments from the skin.
4. Drizzle honey over the top of each grapefruit half.
5. Sprinkle ground cinnamon over the honey.
6. Broil the grapefruit halves for 2-3 minutes or until the honey is caramelized and the grapefruit is slightly browned.
7. Serve the broiled grapefruit halves warm.